# GERIATRIC CHEST DISEASE

# GERIATRIC CHEST DISEASE


LUKE HARRIS

M.B. B.S. (Lond.), M.R.C.P. (Edin.)

*Consultant Chest Physician*
*East Liverpool University Hospital Group*

*Clinical Lecturer in Geriatrics*
*University of Liverpool*



1974
John Wright & Sons Ltd.
Bristol

ISBN 0 7236 0369 3

Printed in Great Britain by John Wright & Sons Ltd. at the Stonebridge Press, Bristol BS4 5NU.

TO MY WIFE AND CHILDREN
IN GRATITUDE FOR THEIR ENCOURAGEMENT

# PREFACE

WE live in an age of specialization and in no sphere is this more evident than in medicine. No physician can nowadays claim, in all honesty, to be fully competent in every field of general (internal) medicine. It is, indeed, difficult for many to keep abreast even of their own speciality, so vast is the output of publications.

Geriatric medicine is the application of general medicine to the elderly, with the addition of particular attention to social needs. The physician practising geriatric medicine, therefore, is in the same predicament as his colleague in general medicine—he cannot know it all.

This, then, explains why I have written this book. It is an attempt to present the Geriatrician, the General Physician and the Chest Physician with a guide to the management of chest disease in the elderly, a subject which has interested me for several years. I have laid emphasis on tempering enthusiasm with humanity both in investigation and treatment, and on the problems of multiple pathology. The views expressed are my own and I have no doubt that some will be disputed. This is in the best tradition of medicine and, if it stimulates refutation by high-quality studies, this is to be welcomed. If the book succeeds simply in interesting others in the problems of geriatric chest disease I will consider the labour to have been worth while.

I would like to acknowledge the help of Miss D. Hawkins in preparing the manuscript and John Wright & Sons Ltd. in the production of the book.

L. H.

# CONTENTS

*Section 1*

# Principles of Diagnosis

*Chapter One*

# Normal Changes in the Ageing Lung

## 1. ANATOMICAL CHANGES

As the lung ages deterioration of tissues ensues, stemming from a variety of causes such as impairment of blood-supply from the bronchial arteries, decreased cell membrane permeability, changes in collagen structure and damage from repeated minor infections: 'fair wear and tear', tobacco and atmospheric pollution.

Autopsy reveals intimal fibrosis of pulmonary vessels, enlarged alveoli (so-called 'senile emphysema'), reduced elastic tissue, thin alveolar walls and decreased pulmonary capillaries, but no increase in total volume of the lungs which deflate normally.

Two other factors influence respiration in relation to age: reduction in the strength of the respiratory muscles and increased stiffness of the thoracic cage.

## 2. PHYSIOLOGICAL CHANGES

Consistent with the autopsy findings there is normal total lung capacity (TLC) in the male, with slight reduction in the female. Vital capacity (VC) decreases with age but residual volume (RV) increases, hence the ratio RV/TLC increases.

The dynamic lung volumes, such as the forced expiratory volume in 1 second ($FEV_1$) or the peak expiratory

Table 1

| Variable | Sex | Height (cm.) 150 | 160 | 170 | 180 | Standard deviation of variable |
|---|---|---|---|---|---|---|
| Vital capacity (VC) (litres) | Males | 2·8 | 3·3 | 3·8 | 4·4 | ±0·6 |
| | Females | 2·0 | 2·4 | 2·8 | 3·3 | ±0·4 |
| Residual volume (RV) (litres) | Males | 1·65 | 2·05 | 2·20 | 2·45 | ±0.55 |
| | Females | 1·65 | 2·05 | 2·20 | 2·45 | ±0·55 |
| Total lung capacity (TLC) (litres) | Males | 4·5 | 5·4 | 6·2 | 7·1 | ±0.9 |
| | Females | 3·6 | 4·4 | 5·1 | 5·7 | ±0·5 |
| Forced expiratory volume in 1 sec. ($FEV_1$) (litres) | Males | 2·0 | 2·2 | 2·6 | 3·0 | ±0·5 |
| | Females | 1·6 | 1·8 | 2·2 | 2·4 | ±0·4 |
| Peak expiratory flow rate (PEFR) (litres per min.) | Males | 430 | 450 | 480 | 510 | ±60 |
| | Females | 290 | 330 | 370 | 410 | ±70 |
| Diffusing capacity (single breath) ($D_L$ or $T_L$) (mm. per min. per mm. Hg) | Males | 21 | 24 | 28 | 31 | ±5 |
| | Females | 20 | 21 | 22 | 23 | ±3 |

| | | | |
|---|---|---|---|
| RV/TLC (per cent) | Males | < 40 | |
| | Females | < 40 | |
| $FEV_1/VC$ (per cent) | Males | 72 | ±11 |
| | Females | 78 | ±9 |
| Physiological dead space ($V_D$) (ml) | Males | 200 | |
| | Females | 200 | |
| Arterial oxygen tension ($Pao_2$) (mm. Hg) | Males | > 75 | |
| | Females | > 75 | |
| Arterial oxygen saturation ($Sao_2$) (per cent) | Males | > 93 | |
| | Females | > 93 | |
| Venous admixture/cardiac output (QS/QT) (per cent) | Males | < 4 | |
| | Females | < 4 | |
| Alveolar–arterial oxygen gradient (A–$aDo_2$) (mm. Hg) | Males | < 30 | |
| | Females | < 30 | |
| Total lung resistance ($R_L$) (cm. $H_2O$ per litre per sec.) | Males | 1·3–4·4 | |
| | Females | 1·3–4·4 | |
| Lung compliance ($C_L$) (litres per cm. $H_2O$) | Males | 0·8–0·23 | |
| | Females | 0·8–0·23 | |

flow rate (PEFR), show a decrease with increasing age. The ratio FEV/VC expressed as a percentage also decreases; forced vital capacity (FVC) is often used in place of VC. Minute ventilation ($\dot{V}_E$) does not appear to be abnormal in the resting state, but is excessive on exercise. Oxygen uptake ($\dot{V}O_2$) is possibly decreased at rest but increased on exercise. This is also shown by the rise in the oxygen ventilation equivalent ($\dot{V}_E/\dot{V}O_2$). Carbon dioxide output ($\dot{V}CO_2$) is probably a little decreased at rest. The ventilatory responses to inhaled $CO_2$ and to 100 per cent $O_2$ are normal. There is some increase in ventilatory dead space.

In the resting state pulmonary arterial pressure, flow and resistance and cardiac output are normal. On exercise, however, maximum cardiac output is decreased. Physiological shunt is increased because of increase in venous admixture effect (i.e., anatomical shunting is not increased).

With increasing age diffusion becomes impaired. The single breath diffusing capacity ($D_L$) or transfer factor ($T_L$) for carbon monoxide decreases with age as does the maximum (exercise) steady-state diffusing capacity.

There are some small changes in blood gases with age. Arterial oxygen tension ($Pa_{O_2}$) and saturation ($Sa_{O_2}$) fall and the alveolar–arterial pressure gradient ($A–aD_{O_2}$) increases. Arterial carbon dioxide tension ($Pa_{CO_2}$) and hydrogen-ion concentration (pH) remain normal.

There are changes in resistance which might be expected, i.e., increase in thoracic and total pulmonary resistance although, strangely airways resistance measured by plethysmography does not appear to be increased (despite the decreases in $FEV_1/FVC$ per cent). Compliance (which is an index of the 'stiffness' of the lungs) is increased, i.e., the lungs are more distensible than in younger persons.

Normal values for these variables are given in Table 1.

*Chapter Two*

# Symptoms

## DYSPNOEA

DYSPNOEA is a subjective sensation, variously described by patients as 'difficulty in breathing', 'shortness of breath', 'short-windedness', 'puffiness', 'inability to catch one's breath', 'smothering', 'choking' and sometimes vaguely 'exhaustion'. It has no direct relationship with measurable respiratory variables such as arterial blood-gas levels or indices of airways resistance. The most convincing explanation of this symptom to date is Campbell's concept of 'inappropriateness'. This implies that dyspnoea is experienced when the individual experiences an increased ventilatory effort which is inappropriate to the result achieved. This is thought to be mediated by length/tension receptors in the respiratory muscles.

In taking a history the following points should be noted:

1. *Onset*: sudden or insidious
2. *Progressive* or *improving*: if improving is it spontaneous or the result of therapy—if so, what?
3. *Rest*: either occurring at rest or relieved by rest
4. *Exercise*: grade of exertional dyspnoea
5. *Industrial exposure*, environmental factors
6. *Associated symptoms*
7. *Smoking* history

A purely clinical approach to the diagnosis of the cause of dyspnoea may have to be made on some occasions. In my experience this is best tackled by considering the main respiratory and cardiac causes in terms of length of history.

## Clinical Analysis

1. SHORT HISTORY
   - *A. Respiratory*
     - i. Pneumonias
     - ii. Spontaneous pneumothorax
     - iii. Inhaled foreign body
   - *B. Cardiac*
     - i. Myocardial infarction
     - ii. Pulmonary embolism
     - iii. Pericardial effusion
     - iv. Left ventricular failure

2. INTERMEDIATE HISTORY (few weeks to few months)
   - *A. Respiratory*
     - i. Pleural effusions
     - ii. Neoplasms
     - iii. Infiltrative conditions
     - iv. Pulmonary tuberculosis
   - *B. Cardiac*
     - i. Congestive cardiac failure
     - ii. Severe anaemias
     - iii. Repeated pulmonary emboli

3. INSIDIOUS ONSET, SLOWLY PROGRESSIVE
     - i. Chronic obstructive lung disease
     - ii. Fibrosing lung diseases

4. OTHER CAUSES
   - *A. Metabolic*
     - i. Diabetes mellitus
     - ii. Uraemia
   - *B. Myasthenia gravis*
   - *C. Psychogenic*

More frequently it will be possible to have a chest X-ray to consider in addition to symptoms and physical signs. It is then possible to adopt a combined approach.

## Clinico-radiological Analysis

1. PAROXYSMAL

*A. Normal X-ray*

i. Bronchial asthma
ii. Ischaemic heart disease (some cases)

*B. Cardiac enlargement*

i. Hypertensive heart disease
ii. Mitral stenosis

2. EXERTIONAL

*A. Normal X-ray*

i. Chronic airways obstruction (some cases)
ii. Primary underventilation
iii. Ankylosing spondylitis
iv. Pulmonary embolism (many cases, if no infarction)
v. Metabolic causes
vi. Severe anaemias

*B. Abnormal X-ray—infiltration*

i. Lymphangitic carcinomatosis
ii. Pulmonary oedema
iii. Sarcoidosis
iv. Pulmonary tuberculosis

*C. Abnormal X-ray—consolidation*

i. Pneumonias
ii. Neoplasms
iii. Pulmonary tuberculosis
iv. Pulmonary infarction

*D. Abnormal X-ray—hypertranslucency*

i. Pneumothorax
ii. Emphysema

*E. Abnormal X-ray—diffuse fibrosis*

i. Fibrosing alveolitis

ii. Pneumoconiosis
iii. Other occupational lung diseases
iv. Pulmonary tuberculosis

*F. Abnormal X-ray—chronic inflammatory changes*

i. Chronic bronchitis (some cases)

When there are facilities available, it is helpful to add a functional approach to the clinical and radiological assessment.

## Functional Analysis

1. FEV/FVC GREATER THAN 70 PER CENT

*A.* $FEV_1$ *and* FVC *normal*

i. Emphysema (some early cases)
ii. Congestive cardiac failure (some mild cases)
iii. Anaemias
iv. Uraemia
v. Diabetes mellitus
vi. Psychogenic

*B.* $FEV_1$ *and* FVC *proportionally reduced* (*'restrictive'*)

i. *Diffusion impaired*
*a.* Fibrosing alveolitis
*b.* Sarcoidosis
*c.* Pneumoconioses

ii. *Diffusion normal*
*a.* Ankylosing spondylitis
*b.* Pleural effusions
*c.* Congestive cardiac failure (some cases)
*d.* Primary alveolar underventilation
*e.* Obesity

2. $FEV_1$/FVC LESS THAN 70 PER CENT ('OBSTRUCTIVE')

*A. Reversible*

i. Bronchial asthma

*B. Irreversible*

i. *Diffusion grossly impaired*
*a.* Emphysema

  *b*. Type A ('emphysematous'), chronic bronchitis
- ii. *Diffusion moderately impaired*
  *a*. Type X ('indeterminate' or 'intermediate') chronic bronchitis
- iii. *Diffusion normal or slightly impaired*
  *a*. Type B ('bronchitic') chronic bronchitis.

From a clinical viewpoint it is useful to classify exertional dyspnoea into grades:

0 = no dyspnoea
1 = dyspnoea on considerable exertion (e.g., stairs)
2 = dyspnoea on moderate exertion (e.g., cannot keep pace with contemporaries on the level)
3 = dyspnoea on mild exertion (e.g., has to stop on level even at own pace)
4 = dyspnoea even at rest

## COUGH

The stimuli which produce cough may be *inflammatory*, e.g., oedema, exudate, ulceration or scarring; *mechanical*, e.g., dusts, smoke (including cigarette smoke which is the commonest cause of cough), foreign bodies or external pressure; *chemical*, e.g., gases, fumes; or *thermal*, e.g., very hot or very cold air.

Although cough may have to be considered purely from a clinical standpoint when of acute onset, it is rare to be unable to obtain a chest X-ray. Indeed it is not an exaggeration to assert that the main diagnostic weapon in the analysis of cough is the chest X-ray and that it is mandatory to have a film taken if a cough persists for more than 3 weeks.

It is nevertheless useful to develop a combined clinico-radiological approach by considering first whether the cough is dry or productive.

## Clinico-radiological Analysis

1. DRY COUGH

*A. Normal X-ray*

i. Upper respiratory tract diseases
ii. Acute bronchitis
iii. Non-opaque foreign bodies, not producing atelectasis
iv. Penduncalated adenoma

*B. Atelectasis*

i. Foreign bodies
ii. Neoplasms
iii. Aneurysms
iv. Glands
v. Mucous plugging

*C. Infiltration*

i. Sarcoidosis
ii. Pulmonary tuberculosis

*D. Diffuse fibrosis*

i. Pneumoconiosis
ii. Fibrosing alveolitis
iii. Pulmonary tuberculosis

*E. Consolidation*

i. Pneumonias (early stages)
ii. Neoplasms
iii. Pulmonary tuberculosis
iv. Pulmonary infarction

2. PRODUCTIVE COUGH

*A. Normal X-ray*

i. Chronic bronchitis (some cases)
ii. Acute bronchitis (later stages)
iii. Bronchiectasis

*B. Consolidation*

i. Pneumonias
ii. Neoplasms
iii. Pulmonary tuberculosis

*C. Cavitation*
- i. Pulmonary tuberculosis
- ii. Neoplasms
- iii. Abscesses
- iv. Mycetoma
- v. Bronchiectasis

*D. Chronic inflammatory*
- i. Chronic bronchitis (some cases)

## HAEMOPTYSIS

Haemoptysis means spitting of blood and may vary from small streaks mixed with saliva or sputum to the expectoration of large quantities of frank blood.

It has to be distinguished from haematemesis which means the vomiting of blood. Usually the distinction is apparent from the history of coughing up as opposed to vomiting up blood. Sometimes, however, it is not clear—especially with an elderly confused patient. In this situation it may be helpful to test the pH, since altered blood from the stomach will in most cases give an acid reaction.

In general any of the conditions which produce cough (q.v.) may be a cause of haemoptysis, and diagnosis may be approached in the same way. It is, however, often useful to consider the most likely causes first.

### Common Causes

1. Chronic bronchitis
2. Neoplasms
3. Pulmonary infarction
4. Pulmonary tuberculosis
5. Bronchiectasis
6. Pneumonias
7. Lung abscess
8. Congestive heart failure
9. Anticoagulant therapy

Other less common causes in the elderly are other respiratory infections, angioma, aneurysm, mitral stenosis, polyarteritis nodosa, blood dyscrasias, etc.

## CHEST PAIN

The complaint of pain in the chest is often difficult to unravel in the elderly patient. The description may be vague, localization may be hazy or the patient may have no clear idea of the time sequence.

It is nevertheless important to try to analyse the symptom—firstly, to try to ascertain the type of pain and, secondly, to consider the causes of each type of pain.

### Analysis of Type

1. ONSET

*A. Acute*

i. Pulmonary embolism
ii. Spontaneous pneumothorax
iii. Myocardial infarction
iv. Angina pectoris
v. Dissecting aneurysm.

*B. Insidious*

2. SITE

*A. Central, substernal* +/− radiation to neck, down one or both arms and sometimes to jaw or between shoulder-blades = *cardiac pain* usually, but may be mimicked by oesophageal pain

*B. Localized*

i. Nerve-root distribution
ii. Point of shoulder—suggests diaphragmatic involvement
iii. Rib or vertebra—suggests local pathology
iv. Other distribution—suggests pleural involvement

3. PERIODICITY
   *A. Constant*
      i. Bone pain
      ii. Aneurysm
      iii. Neoplasm
   *B. Intermittent—short periods*
      i. Angina pectoris
      ii. Hiatus hernia
      iii. Pleurisy
   *C. Intermittent—long periods*
      i. Myocardial infarction
      ii. Referred pain from peptic ulcer or gall bladder disease

4. CHARACTER
   *A. Constricting* = cardiac (but sometimes bronchospasm associated with similar description)
   *B. Stabbing* = pleuritic
   *C. Burning* = oesophageal
   *D. Soreness* = tracheobronchial

5. AGGRAVATING FACTORS
   *A. Breathing* = pleuritic
   *B. Movement* = root pain
   *C. Yawning, sneezing, coughing* = root pain, pleurisy
   *D. During eating* = oesophageal or gastric
   *E. During exercise* = angina
   *F. After exercise* = effort syndrome

6. RELIEVING FACTORS
   *A. Rest* = angina
   *B. Immobilization* = pleurisy or rib fracture
   *C. Alkali* = peptic ulceration
   *D. Trinitrin* = angina (usually) or oesophageal (occasionally)
   *E. Beta-adrenergic stimulant* = bronchospasm
   *F. Beta-adrenergic blocker* = angina

7. ASSOCIATED SYMPTOMS
   A. *Cough, sputum, haemoptysis*—suggests respiratory cause
   B. *Palpitations*—suggests effort syndrome
   C. *Vomiting, nausea, anorexia*—suggests oesophageal or gastric cause
   D. *Dyspnoea, wheezing*—may be either respiratory or cardiac

Having established the type of pain as far as possible the underlying causes can be considered in a systematic manner, with ancillary investigations of which chest X-ray and electrocardiogram are basic.

## Causes

1. RESPIRATORY
   A. *Pleural*
      i. Tuberculous
      ii. Pulmonary infarction
      iii. Neoplasm
      iv. Spontaneous pneumothorax
      v. Rheumatoid disease
   B. *Tracheobronchial*
      i. Bronchitis
      ii. Neoplasm
   C. *Diaphragmatic*
      i. Diaphragmatic pleurisy
      ii. Bornholm disease

2. CARDIOVASCULAR
   A. *Angina*
   B. *Myocardial infarction*
   C. *Syphilitic aortic aneurysm*
   D. *Dissecting aneurysm*
   E. *Pericarditis*

3. MEDIASTINAL
   A. *Oesophageal*
      i. Hiatus hernia
      ii. Peptic ulcer
      iii. Neoplasm
      iv. Oesophagitis
   B. *Neoplastic*
      i. Bronchial carcinoma
      ii. Reticulosis
      iii. Secondary malignant glands

4. SPINAL
   A. *Cervical spondylosis and disc lesions*
   B. *Secondary deposits in vertebrae*
   C. *Tuberculosis of vertebrae*
   D. *Myelomatosis*
   E. *Osteo-arthritis of thoracic spine*
   F. *Osteoporosis of thoracic spine*
   G. *Osteomalacia of thoracic spine*
   H. *Pressure from aneurysm*

5. CHEST WALL
   A. *Herpes zoster*
   B. *Intercostal neuralgia*
   C. *Breast pathology*
   D. *Secondary deposits in ribs*
   E. *Myalgia*
   F. *Pressure on ribs from aneurysm*

6. PSYCHOGENIC
   A. *Effort syndrome (cardiac neurosis)*

7. REFERRED FROM ABDOMEN
   A. *Gall-bladder disease*
   B. *Gastric ulcer*
   C. *Subphrenic abscess*

It is often possible to proceed a considerable way towards diagnosis and reduce the extent of investigation by considering, in the first instance, the commoner causes of chest pain in the elderly.

### Common Causes

1. EXERCISE-INDUCED
   *A. Angina pectoris*

2. BREATHING-RELATED
   *A. Pleurisy*
      i. Neoplasm
      ii. Pneumonia
      iii. Pulmonary infarction

3. POSTURE-RELATED
   *A. Oesophageal*
      i. Hiatus hernia
   *B. Vertebral*
      i. Cervical spondylosis or osteo-arthritis
      ii. Thoracic osteo-arthritis
      iii. Thoracic osteoporosis

4. OCCURRING AT REST
   *A. Myocardial infarction*
   *B. Bony metastases*

It should be remembered that chronic bronchitics often complain of substernal pain (= soreness) after coughing, and sometimes on exercise (as the result of increased coughing produced by exertion), which should not be confused with true angina pectoris.

## SPUTUM

### Clinical Examination

Sputum is produced by the same stimuli as those which are responsible for cough (q.v.). Normally the bronchial mucosa produces 100 ml. of mucus in each 24 hours. This is distributed as a blanket about 5 μm. thick which is moved upwards from bronchi to trachea and then further upwards until it tips over into the oesophagus. If excess mucus is produced the normal process of removal is insufficient leading to accumulation of mucus and the production of sputum.

## Diagnostic Significance

1. QUANTITY

A. *Copious* (more than 150 ml. per day)
- i. Bronchiectasis
- ii. Acute pulmonary oedema
- iii. Lung abscess
- iv. Bronchopleural fistula
- v. Extensive cavitating pulmonary tuberculosis

B. *Moderate* (10–100 ml. per day)
- i. Chronic bronchitis
- ii. Other pulmonary infections

C. *Scanty* (less than 10 ml. per day)
- i. Pulmonary emphysema
- ii. Early stages of acute tracheobronchial and pulmonary infections

2. COLOUR

A. *White (or clear)* = mucoid
B. *Yellow* = fresh pus
C. *Green* = stale pus
D. *Black* = carbon or changed blood
E. *Brown* = changed blood
F. *Pink* = blood-tinged oedema fluid
G. *Red streaks* = fresh blood
H. *Portions of green or yellow in white background* = mucopurulent

3. ODOUR
   *A. Foul*
      i. Lung abscess
      ii. Bronchiectasis

4. CONSISTENCY
   *A. Sticky*
      i. Infection
      ii. Mucoid sputum in chronic bronchitis
   *B. Frothy*
      i. Pulmonary oedema
      ii. Bronchitis

*Chapter Three*

# Physical Signs

A COMPLETE account of all the physical signs possible in disease of the respiratory system would be out of place here. Instead the main clinical causes of the most important physical signs are summarized.

## MAIN PHYSICAL SIGNS—CLINICAL CAUSES

### 1. IMPAIRED PERCUSSION

*A*. Consolidation
*B*. Effusion ('stony' dullness)
*C*. Atelectasis (collapse)
*D*. Fibrosis
*E*. Pleural thickening
*F*. Elevated hemidiaphragm
*G*. Neoplasm (large)

### 2. BRONCHIAL BREATHING

*A*. Consolidation
*B*. Shallow effusion
*C*. Collapse of peripheral lung parenchyma with patent major bronchus
*D*. Large cavity near surface
*E*. Pneumothorax (occasionally; more often there is silence)

## 3. CRACKLES (crepitations)

These sounds are *not* due to air bubbling through fluid but a result of the opening (inspiratory) or closing (expiratory) of abnormal alveoli, i.e., alveoli which have been rendered more rigid (less compliant) by pathological processes such as oedema, fibrosis etc.

*A.* Pneumonias
*B.* Bronchitis
*C.* Bronchiectasis
*D.* Tuberculosis
*E.* Left ventricular failure
*F.* Fibrosis (especially fibrosing alveolitis)

## 4. WHEEZING

Wheezing is produced by narrowing of bronchi. The mechanism of production of these abnormal sounds is like that of a reed instrument. The walls of the narrowed bronchus come into close approximation and vibration produces the sounds which are musical in character. The pitch of the sounds is dependent on the velocity of air flow and does not therefore indicate the size or calibre of the bronchi involved. Most wheezes, in fact, appear to arise from the larger rather than the smaller bronchi. Wheezes are much more frequently expiratory than inspiratory because there is, even normally, a reduction in calibre during expiration.

UNDERLYING PATHOLOGY

*A. Bronchial wall*
- i. Bronchospasm—asthma, bronchial and cardiac
- ii. Stricture
  - *a.* Bronchiectasis
  - *b.* Neoplasm

*B. Bronchial lumen*
- i. Secretions
- ii. Tumours

*C. Bronchial mucosa*
- i. Oedema
  - *a.* Infections
  - *b.* Chemical and physical irritants
  - *c.* Allergy
  - *d.* Left ventricular failure

*D. External compression*
- i. Tumours (may give localized wheeze, heard only in certain positions)
- ii. Aortic aneurysm

The reversibility of wheezing can be assessed by the administration of a bronchodilator. This can be done on a clinical basis by simple auscultation, but frequently this is not adequate for the obstruction (except in 'pure' asthma) will usually be only partially reversed. It is better therefore to measure the effect on the $FEV_1$, taking a 20 per cent increase over the basal reading as indicating a significant degree of reversibility. It is also necessary to test the effects of the different classes of bronchodilator (β-2-adrenergic stimulant, metaxanthine, atropine) and corticosteroid before concluding that the condition is irreversible.

Apart from the above-mentioned mechanisms, there are a number of factors which may precipitate wheezing, i.e., exercise, thermal changes in ambient conditions, allergenic exposure.

## 5. DIFFUSE AIRWAYS OBSTRUCTION

*A.* Generalized wheezing
*B.* Little or no chest expansion
*C.* Use of accessory muscles of respiration
*D.* Indrawing of costal margin on inspiration
*E.* Loss of cardiac and/or hepatic dullness
*F.* Shortening of the trachea (in normals it is possible to fit the breadth of three fingers between the cricothyroid and the suprasternal notch)

*G.* Tracheal tug (related to respiration, not to heart beat)
*H.* Prolonged expiration (forced expiratory time (FET) more than 6 sec.)
*I.* Jugular venous engorgement during expiration

*Chapter Four*

# Laboratory Evaluation

## 1. CHEST X-RAY

WHENEVER possible previous chest X-rays should be obtained for comparison with the current film, as this will help evaluate whether changes are recent or chronic.

In purely practical terms the chest X-ray should be considered an essential part of examination of the respiratory system—it is virtually an extension of inspection. Frequently it will serve as a short cut or at least a useful signpost.

For a full exposition of chest radiology it is necessary to refer to standard works on the subject. Here it is reasonable to give only a summary of some of the more important findings.

### Summary of Major Abnormalities

*A.* LARGE HOMOGENEOUS OPACITIES

- i. Effusion
- ii. Atelectasis
- iii. Consolidation

*B.* CIRCULAR OPACITIES

- i. Neoplasms—primary or secondary, benign or malignant
- ii. Granulomata—including tuberculosis
- iii. Infections
- iv. Pulmonary infarcts

*C.* DIFFUSE NODULAR OPACITIES

i. Infections
ii. Pneumoconioses
iii. Fibrosing alveolitis
iv. Pulmonary oedema
v. Sarcoidosis
vi. Collagenoses
vii. Reticuloses
viii. Lymphangitic carcinomatasis
ix. Allergies

*D.* LINEAR SHADOWS

i. Pleural
ii. Lymphatic
iii. Fibrotic
iv. Atelactatic
v. Pulmonary infarcts (healed)

*E.* RING SHADOWS ('CAVITIES')

i. Emphysematous bullae
ii. Cavities
    *a.* Tuberculous
    *b.* Neoplastic
    *c.* Staphylococcal and other infections (abscess)

*F.* HONEYCOMB SHADOWING

i. Fibrosing alveolitis
ii. Systemic sclerosis
iii. Pneumoconioses (some)
iv. Lymphangitic carcinomatosis
v. Bronchiectasis
vi. Pulmonary congestion (cardiac failure)

*G.* HIGH-DENSITY SHADOWS

i. Calcified tuberculous lesions
ii. Certain dusts—Fe, Ba, Sn, Ca
iii. Opaque foreign bodies

*H.* INCREASED TRANSLUCENCY

i. Pneumothorax
ii. Emphysema
iii. Hiatus hernia (stomach gas)

*I.* BONY LESIONS

i. Metastases
ii. Erosions
iii. Fractures

## 2. BRONCHOGRAPHY

The value of bronchography lies in:

*A.* Confirming or excluding bronchiectasis;
*B.* Localizing the site of or demonstrating the presence of a bronchial block.

Its main indication is in the investigation of unexplained haemoptysis or an incompletely resolved pneumonia or other indeterminate shadows (especially those beyond the reach of a bronchoscope).

It is debatable, however, whether this investigation is justified in the elderly. It is at best an unpleasant procedure from which fatalities or near-fatalities may occur from time to time. No surgeon will operate for bronchiectasis in an elderly patient, and few will resect a carcinoma in a patient once the patient has reached the age of 70. In most instances, therefore, it would be a purely academic investigation and not in the patient's interest.

## 3. TOMOGRAPHY

This is a most useful additional radiological investigation for:

*A.* Demonstration of cavities
*B.* Segmental localization
*C.* Elucidation of abnormal shadows

*D.* Demonstrations of the lumen of trachea and larger bronchi
*E.* Demonstration of hilar gland enlargement
*F.* Demonstration of pulmonary vasculature

## 4. SPUTUM

### A. Smear

i. Gram stain for non-tuberculous organisms (NTO)
ii. Ziehl-Neelsen stain for tubercle bacilli
iii. Asbestos bodies

### B. Cytology

i. Malignant cells
ii. Eosinophils—allergies

### C. Culture (and sensitivity tests)

i. Tubercle
ii. Other pathogens (NTO)

If sputum is not obtainable, bacteriology may be performed on laryngeal swabs or gastric washings.

## 5. SKIN TESTS

### A. Tuberculin Test

Often negative in very old or seriously debilitated patients.

### B. Kveim Test

An important test in the diagnosis of sarcosis.

### C. Hypersensitivity Tests for Allergy

i. House dust and house-dust mite
ii. *Aspergillus*
iii. Many others, pollen, animal hair, etc.

} not often indicated in the elderly

### D. Specific Tests for Various Fungi, Hydatid, Brucella, etc.

## 6. LARYNGOSCOPY

For demonstrating recurrent laryngeal palsy (hoarseness).

## 7. BRONCHOSCOPY

This procedure is of value in the diagnosis of bronchial carcinoma:

i. To visualize the neoplasm
ii. To take a biopsy specimen
iii. To aspirate secretions for cytological examination

There are a number of contra-indications to the procedure in the elderly:

*A.* Cardiac disease—especially arrythmias
*B.* Chronic respiratory failure
*C.* When bleeding might cause fatal occlusion, e.g., adenoma, bronchostenosis
*D.* Age over 70 (in the view of most surgeons)
*E.* $FEV_1$ less than 1 litre
*F.* Other serious disease, e.g., neurological, endocrine, etc.

## 8. BIOPSY

### A. Pleural

This is a relatively easy procedure using the Abrams needle, and not really distressing if adequate local anaesthesia is employed. It is usually carried out at the same time as pleural aspiration and should be performed only if fluid is present. Although the biopsy samples are small there is a sufficiently high incidence of positive findings for malignancy and tuberculosis to make it well worth while and worth repeating if necessary.

### B. Lung

Lung biopsy may be performed as open biopsy by a chest surgeon (with the same contra-indications as for bronchoscopy) or as needle biopsy using a high-powered drill. The main indications are for diagnosis of a solid tumour or the nature of a diffuse fibrosis. Needle biopsy may save the patient a needless thoracotomy, e.g., oat-cell carcinoma, although there is some risk of producing a pneumothorax. In the case of a diffuse fibrosis, it would be a purely academic exercise in an elderly patient since, if it were a form amenable to any treatment, the only treatment available would be the administration of corticosteroid (which would be given as a therapeutic trial anyway).

### C. Lymph Nodes—Superficial

This is generally a fairly simple procedure which may give a histological diagnosis in sarcoidosis, malignancy, reticuloses, or tuberculosis (rarely in the elderly).

### D. Lymph Nodes—Mediastinal

This procedure, which is carried out by a surgeon skilled in the technique, has been reported to be of great value in some centres. It permits biopsy of nodes otherwise inaccessible except by thoracotomy. The major hazards are pneumothorax and bleeding.

## 9. SEROLOGY AND BIOCHEMISTRY

There are a number of serological and biochemical tests which may be of value in diagnosis. Some of the more important are listed below.

### A. Rheumatoid Factor

Positive in some cases of fibrosing alveolitis

### B. Antinuclear Factor and L.E. Cells

Positive in many cases of systemic lupus erythematosus

**C. Agglutination Tests**

Positive for specific viruses

**D. Precipitin Tests**

Positive in bronchopulmonary aspergillosis and some forms of fibrosing alveolitis (e.g., 'bird-fancier's lung.)

**E. Alpha-antitrypsin**

May be reduced in some cases of 'pure' emphysema, especially of lower lobes, and with a genetic basis.

**F. Serum Calcium**

Raised in some cases of sarcoidosis

**G. Serum Gamma-globulin**

Increased in:

i. Chronic infections
ii. Collagenoses
iii. Sarcoidosis
iv. Lymphomas
v. Myelomatosis

**H. Serum Transaminases**

i. Normal serum glutamic oxalo-acetic acid transaminase (SGOT) and serum glutamic pyruvic transaminase (SGPT) with raised lactic dehydrogenase (LDH) in some cases of pulmonary infarction
ii. Raised SGOT and SGPT early with late rise in LDH in myocardial infarction

**I. Full Blood Picture**

May show evidence of a haematological process contributing to the condition, e.g., polycythaemia, anaemia, leukaemia, leucocytosis, etc.

**J. Erythrocyte Sedimentation Rate**

Often very high in malignancy and myelomatosis

## 10. ELECTROCARDIOGRAPHY

An electrocardiogram may provide useful information in any patient with respiratory symptoms.

### A. Right Ventricular Hypertrophy (Pulmonary Hypertension)

The diagnostic findings are a dominant R wave over the right ventricle ($V_4R$, $V_3R$, $V_1$) followed by T-wave inversion. Other ECG findings may be suggestive but *not* pathognomonic, e.g., dominant S wave in $V_5$, P pulmonale.

### B. Left Ventricular Hypertrophy

The diagnostic findings are R wave in $V_5$ greater than 25 mV. or R in $V_5$ plus S in $V_1$ greater than 35 mV. Other findings such as T-wave inversion may support the diagnosis.

### C. Myocardial Ischaemia

In the acute phase there will be S–T segment depression in some leads with reciprocal elevation in others depending on the site of the infarct. In the chronic phases there will be T-wave inversion (of symmetrical shape) in the appropriate leads, or there may be a planar type of S–T depression. Such changes may be absent at rest and require exercise to reveal them.

### D. Acute Pulmonary Embolism

The classical findings are a deep S in lead I, a pathological Q in lead III (followed by T-wave inversion) and T-wave inversion over the right ventricule. Arrhythmias may occur but are not diagnostic.

## 11. ANGIOGRAPHY

This is a method of demonstrating the anatomy of the pulmonary vasculature and the sites of any obstruction.

## 12. LUNG SCANNING

The lungs are scanned by a scintillation counter after intravenous administration of micro-aggregates of human albumin labelled with a radioactive isotope (usually technetium-99). This is a good method of demonstrating perfusion defects due to pulmonary emboli, but must be carefully interpreted in relation to any abnormal shadows seen on the chest X-ray, e.g., an area of fibrosis will show diminished perfusion.

## 13. RESPIRATORY FUNCTION TESTS

### A. At Rest

Much information can be obtained from a few tests which require only a little co-operation from the patient (although this is sometimes impossible to obtain in the elderly deaf or confused patient).

#### i. TIMED SPIROMETRY

The basic manœuvre is to record a tracing during forced expiration after a maximum inspiration. From this tracing the forced expiratory volume in the first second ($FEV_1$) and the forced vital capacity (FVC) can be measured. The relationship between the two indices is important in distinguishing between 'obstructive' and 'restrictive' lung disease. If the ratio $FEV_1/FVC$ is less than 70 per cent in an elderly subject there is expiratory airways obstruction present. If the ratio is greater than 70 per cent, but the absolute values are less than 80 per cent of predicted (Table 1) there is restriction of respiration present.

Other measurements from the tracing may possibly be more sensitive indicators of the degree of obstruction (once this has been established) but do not distinguish the two types of ventilatory impairment. These measures, such as the maximum mid-expiratory flow rate, are also more laborious to calculate.

Similarly, the peak flow rate (PFR) which, is easy to measure on a cheap readily portable apparatus, does not differentiate between 'obstructive' and 'restrictive'. It is, however, a useful instrument for overall assessment of ventilatory impairment, particularly for follow-up purposes.

ii. BLOOD GASES

The measurement of arterial oxygen tension and carbon dioxide tension is probably the most important lung-function estimate of all, since respiration is, by definition, that process resulting in oxygenation of the mixed venous blood and elimination of excess carbon dioxide.

Without going deeply into mechanisms and concepts of respiratory physiology it may be said that there are two main types of respiratory failure: hypoxaemia alone and hypoxaemia with carbon dioxide retention. Hypoxaemia alone may result from any respiratory disease or from cardiac disease. Hypoxaemia with hypercapnia indicates generalized underventilation (or more accurately generalized lowering of ventilation/perfusion ratios). Blood gases can be measured on arterial samples or on 'arterialized' capillary samples. Carbon dioxide tension can be estimated by a bloodless rebreathing method which gives a measurement of the oxygenated mixed venous $Pco_2$ (average 6 mm. Hg more than arterial).

iii. DIFFUSION AND TOTAL LUNG CAPACITY

The measurement of diffusing capacity (or transfer factor) is of value in the diagnosis of emphysema and of the diffuse fibroses, in both of which it is reduced. It is desirable, therefore, to relate diffusing capacity to lung volume. This is usually done by a separate measurement of lung volume. In emphysema there will be an increased total lung capacity whereas in a diffuse fibrosis there will be reduced total lung capacity.

However, if the relationship of diffusion to the alveolar volume at which the measurement was made is considered, it no longer becomes necessary to have a separate assessment of total capacity.

This relationship ($D_L/V_A$) is the diffusion coefficient (sometimes called *k*CO) and is easily and rapidly performed with modern automated equipment (provided the patient can hold his breath for 10 sec.). The ratio is greatly reduced in emphysema and is associated with an 'obstructive' pattern. In the diffuse fibrosis *k*CO is reduced and associated with a 'restrictive' pattern.

These tests will by and large provide the answers to the disturbances of function in the majority of patients. There are, of course, many other tests which may be carried out when more detailed assessment is required.

## B. On Exercise

Limitation of exercise tolerance may be a manifestation of various disease processes. In the assessment of disability, the elucidation of underlying systemic disease, the measurement of response to therapy and subsequent progress, it is desirable to quantify the patient's exercise tolerance. A number of factors are concerned in the ability to perform physical work, e.g., cardiac, respiratory, locomotor, and they may be affected separately and tested individually. In many cases, however, it is the integration of these systems that breaks down and disease in one system may manifest itself by its effect on another system.

Some of the methods which are practicable in assessing exercise tolerance in the elderly are indicated below.

### i. QUALITATIVE

#### *a. HISTORY*

Assessment based on the patient's history provides at best a rough guide to disability, since the threshold for dyspnoea, pain or exhaustion differs from one individual to another. In addition, there is always the difficulty of obtaining a satisfactory history from some elderly patients because of such factors as loss of memory, vagueness or confusion. Nevertheless, there is some value in grading the symptoms thus:

0 = absence of symptom
1 = occurs on considerable exertion
2 = occurs on moderate exertion
3 = occurs on mild exertion
4 = occurs at rest

A change of grade usually indicates a definite improvement or deterioration. This grading may be applied to many symptoms, e.g., dyspnoea, angina, palpitation, exhaustion, intermittent claudication, etc.

*b. DIRECT OBSERVATION*

It is at times not at all clear which symptom is limiting exercise, especially when the complaint is of 'exhaustion' or 'weakness'. Under such circumstances, if the physician accompanies the patient along the corridor and up the stairs he can see whether exercise is halted by pain or dyspnoea, muscle fatigue or palpitation, locomotor or neurological disability.

ii. QUANTITATIVE

In quantitative testing of exercise tolerance the general principle of testing to near maximum ability should be adopted, not only to discover the patient's maximum work capacity but also because failure of adaptation may not be apparent at minimal work loads. This often necessitates measurements at two or three work loads.

Exercise may be performed on a small set of steps. The work can be varied by altering the rate of stepping and the height of the steps. This is the cheapest apparatus but has the disadvantages that only moderate work loads can be obtained, electrocardiographic monitoring is rendered difficult and is unsuitable for patients with vertigo, etc. More sophisticated methods are the use of a treadmill or a bicycle ergometer. Both are much more expensive than steps but have certain advantages. The treadmill is much nearer to the patient's everyday activities while the bicycle ergometer can be adjusted for arm exercise when there is lower limb disability, and certain tests are much more easily performed with a patient sitting on a bicycle, e.g., blood-pressure measurements, blood samples.

The work load for the step test is calculated as

$$\text{Work} = \text{height of step (metres)} \times \text{frequency (steps per minute)} \times \text{weight (kg.)}$$

and is expressed as kg. m. per min. Treadmill work is related to body-weight, speed of the treadmill and its incline. Work on the bicycle ergometer is measured in kg. m. per min. (or kp. m. per min.) or in watts, depending on the restraint imposed on the flywheel.

Since the various forms of exercise are not strictly equivalent even when the external work is equal, it is better to record the energy expenditure in terms of oxygen consumption in the elderly.

### *a. EXERCISE VENTILATION, HEART-RATE AND ELECTROCARDIOGRAM*

Exercise ventilation ($\dot{V}_E$ in litres per min.) is easily measured with a Wright respiratory anemometer or a Parkinson-Cowen dry gas meter. The measurement is usually made during the fifth or sixth minute of exercise by which time a (relatively) steady state has been reached. Electrocardiographic monitoring is carried out throughout. Heart-rate is determined from the tracings. If S–T changes or arrhythmias occur exercise is terminated. An immediate post-exercise full ECG is recorded to look for ischaemic changes.

An isolated measurement of $\dot{V}_E$ or exercise heart-rate is of limited value, but repeated measurements over a period of time for follow-up purposes are more informative. Measurements obtained may be compared with the normal ranges given in Table 2.

*b. OXYGEN VENTILATION EQUIVALENT*

It requires only a little more effort to measure the oxygen consumption ($\dot{V}O_2$ litres per min.). The simplest and cheapest apparatus are a Douglas bag, a low-resistance one-way valve and a Lloyd-Haldane or a micro-Scholander apparatus for oxygen analysis. These chemical analyses, however, require considerable manual dexterity and practice; a slightly more expensive paramagnetic $O_2$ analyser obviates this difficulty.

The oxygen ventilation equipment is then calculated as $V_E/\dot{V}O_2$: in elderly men the upper limit is 35 and in elderly women 30. A higher figure indicates an excessive ventilatory response.

In calculating $O_2$ consumption a correction must be made for any change in volume resulting from the difference between volume of carbon dioxide evolved and volume of oxygen taken up.

$$\dot{V}O_2 = \dot{V}_E \times [(F_IO_2 \times F_EN_2/F_IN_2) - F_EO_2] \times K,$$

where

$F_IO_2$ = inspired $O_2$ concentration as a fraction (i.e., 0·2093),

$F_IN_2$ = inspired $N_2$ concentration as a fraction (i.e., 0·7904),

$F_EO_2$ = expired $O_2$ concentration as a fraction,

$F_EN_2$ = expired $N_2$ concentration as a fraction = $1 - (F_EO_2 + F_ECO_2)$ where $F_ECO_2$ = concentration of expired $CO_2$,

K = factor for conversion to STPD.

Table 2—Normal values for some cardiorespiratory variables at three levels of exercise in elderly subjects

| Sex | Exercise grade | Step test: Height (cm.) | Step test: Rate (steps per min.) | kp. m. per min. (or kg. m. per min.) | Watts | Oxygen consumption (litres per min.) ($\dot{V}O_2$) |
|---|---|---|---|---|---|---|
| Men | Mild | 20 | 15 | 200 | 35 | 1·0 |
| | Moderate | 25 | 23 | 400 | 70 | 1·5 |
| | Severe | 30 | 29 | 600 | 150 | 2·0 |
| Women | Mild | 20 | 13 | 150 | 25 | 0·8 |
| | Moderate | 25 | 20 | 300 | 50 | 1·0 |
| | Severe | 30 | 25 | 450 | 75 | 1·5 |

| Sex | Exercise grade | Carbon dioxide output (litres per min.) ($\dot{V}CO_2$) | Minute ventilation (litres per min.) ($\dot{V}_E$) | Cardiac output (litres per min.) ($\dot{Q}_t$) | Heart-rate (cycles per min.) | Oxygen ventilation equivalent (litres per litre) ($V_E/\dot{V}O_2$) |
|---|---|---|---|---|---|---|
| Men | Mild | 0·9 | $25 \pm 5$ | $11 \pm 2$ | 100 | $< 35$ |
| | Moderate | 1·5 | $40 \pm 5$ | $15 \pm 3$ | 130 | $< 35$ |
| | Severe | 2·0 | $70 \pm 15$ | $20 \pm 3$ | 150 | $< 35$ |
| Women | Mild | 0·7 | $20 \pm 5$ | $10 \pm 4$ | 100 | $< 30$ |
| | Moderate | 1·0 | $35 \pm 5$ | $13 \pm 3$ | 130 | $< 30$ |
| | Severe | 1·5 | $55 \pm 10$ | $15 \pm 4$ | 150 | $< 30$ |

*c. CARDIAC OUTPUT (INDIRECT FICK $CO_2$ METHOD)*
Cardiac output ($\dot{Q}_t$ litres per min.) can be measured during exercise by the indirect Fick $CO_2$ method which states that

$$\dot{Q}_t = \dot{V}co_2/(C\bar{v}co_2 - Caco_2),$$

where

$$C\bar{v}co_2 = CO_2 \text{ content in mixed venous blood,}$$
$$Caco_2 = CO_2 \text{ content in arterial blood,}$$
$$\dot{V}co_2 = CO_2 \text{ expired in litres per min.}$$

This entails analysis of expired air for $CO_2$, measurement of mixed venous carbon dioxide tension by the rebreathing method, and measurement of arterial carbon dioxide tension. Carbon dioxide contents are then derived from McHardy's tables (1967).

*A*. $CO_2$ output is obtained by analysis of expired air. Measurement of minute volume ($\dot{V}co_2 = \dot{V}_E \times F_Eco_2$). The Lloyd-Haldane or micro-Scholander apparatus can be used for this at the same time as for oxygen. If $\dot{V}o_2$ is not required it is easier to use the Campbell-Howell half-Haldane apparatus.

*B*. Mixed venous $CO_2$ tension is derived from the rebreathing $Pco_2$. The method and correction factors were fully described by Jones and others (1967) and anyone proposing to use the method should refer to the original paper. The technique necessitates the use of an infra-red rapid $CO_2$ analyser which is a relatively expensive piece of equipment. It can, of course, be used for all $CO_2$ gas-phase measurements.

*C*. Arterial $CO_2$ pressure ($Paco_2$) may be obtained by taking blood samples from the hyperaemic ear lobe into heparinized capillary tubes. A correction factor of + 2·5 mm. Hg is added to the ear-lobe value to correct it to arterial value on exercise. Naturally it is necessary to have facilities for blood-gas analysis for such studies.

Results obtained by this method correlate well with dye-dilution methods. Normal limits for cardiac output in the elderly are given in Table 2.

*d. ARTERIAL BLOOD GASES*

Both $Po_2$ and $Pco_2$ can be measured with modern blood-gas analysers, either on arterial samples or 'arterialized' ear-lobe samples.

In normal subjects there is usually little rise in $Pco_2$ and no change in $Po_2$ on even moderate exercise. A rise in $Pco_2$ of more than 5 mm. Hg implies that a ventilatory limit has been reached (i.e., the metabolic load is greater than can be dealt with by respiratory mechanisms). A fall in $Po_2$ greater than 5 mm. Hg implies a defect of diffusion (or pulmonary transfer of oxygen) such as may occur in diffuse fibrotic conditions (e.g., fibrosing alveolitis) or in pure emphysema.

The alveolar–arterial oxygen gradient can be calculated from the data previously obtained in the studies outlined above. Alveolar oxygen tension ($P_Ao_2$) can be obtained as a very close approximation for clinical purposes from the equation:

$$P_Ao_2 = P_Io_2 - Paco_2/R,$$

where

$$R = \dot{V}co_2/\dot{V}o_2,$$

$$P_Io_2 = 0{\cdot}2093 \times (P_B - 47)$$

where

$$P_B = \text{atmospheric pressure in mm. Hg.}$$

The alveolar–arterial gradient ($A\text{–}aDo_2$) is obtained by subtraction.

In the elderly the upper limit of normal is 35 mm. Hg during exercise. A widening of the gradient on exercise implies a worsening of ventilation-perfusion relationships, i.e., ventilation is inadequate in relation to the increased cardiac output.

### iii. RELATIONSHIP TO EVERYDAY ACTIVITIES

#### *a. MILD EXERCISE*

In terms of energy requirements the following may be considered as forms of mild exercise: sewing, dusting, washing, painting, driving a car, eating and slow walking.

#### *b. MODERATE EXERCISE*

Similarly in relation to energy expenditure, moderate exercise is provided by: dancing (old time), fast walking, golf, swimming, bowling, ironing, bedmaking, clothes washing and climbing stairs.

#### *c. SEVERE EXERCISE*

Severe exercise involves activities such as running or skating in which comparatively few elderly people indulge.

*Section 2*

# Specific Diseases

*Chapter Five*

# Chronic Airways Obstruction

FEW elderly patients present with simple chronic bronchitis, pure emphysema or uncomplicated asthma. On the other hand, combinations of chronic bronchitis with varying degrees of emphysema with or without asthma are common. Thus, in an analysis of 500 consecutive patients over the age of 65 admitted under my care for respiratory symptoms, 42 per cent of the men and 26 per cent of the women were suffering from chronic bronchitis and its complications (excluding frank bronchopneumonia). Chronic airways obstruction is a convenient term for describing the end-state of these three major obstructive conditions (*see* Table 3).

In discussing this group of diseases some definition of terms is desirable for there is much confusion in the literature.

Chronic bronchitis is primarily a clinical diagnosis, i.e., a syndrome of cough with sputum for at least 3 months of the year in 2 successive years in the absence of other causes for the symptoms. The pathological basis is excessive production of mucus in response to irritants such as cigarette smoke, air pollutants and infection. Note that dyspnoea is not an essential feature of the diagnosis although it is a common sequel of the condition.

Emphysema is primarily a pathological diagnosis, i.e., demonstrable increase in size of air-spaces distal to the terminal bronchi (Reid 1967). Note that destruction of alveoli is not an essential feature of the diagnosis, as this would exclude atrophic and hypoplastic forms of emphysema. Emphysema may be diagnosed with reasonable accuracy in some cases by radiography, i.e., hypertranslucency due to diminished vascularity (this is the only criterion which correlates with autopsy findings). Emphysema may also be diagnosed by certain physiological tests, i.e., a raised total lung capacity in association with a marked reduction of diffusing capacity (transfer factor).

Asthma is primarily a functional definition, i.e., expiratory airways obstruction which is reversible either spontaneously or as a result of therapy. Note that the definition does not include any speculation about possible allergens nor does it define reversibility. In practice, however, reversibility implies at least 20 per cent increase in $FEV_1$ over the basal level following administration of a bronchodilator. A chronic state with exacerbation and remissions but never remitting to completely normal function is also included by the definition.

Subdivisions of the 'chronic bronchitic syndrome' have been proposed on a combination of clinical, physiological and radiological features. These subdivisions seem to be dependent upon the degree of emphysema associated with the chronic bronchitis, at one extreme being patients with severe emphysema and only mild bronchitis while at the other extreme are patients with severe bronchitis and little or no emphysema.

1. The *emphysematous* type (Type A, 'pink puffers') show:

*A.* Dyspnoea often appears disproportionately severe
*B.* Sputum less than 10 ml. per day
*C.* Slight reduction in $Po_2$ (not cyanosed)
*D.* Low or normal $Pco_2$
*E.* Vascular deficit on chest X-ray
*F.* Considerably reduced diffusing capacity and *k*CO with raised total lung capacity

2. The *bronchitic* type (Type B, 'blue bloaters') show:
*A*. Cough and sputum (more than 10 ml. per day)
*B*. Mild to severe reduction in $Po_2$ (often sufficient to produce cyanosis)
*C*. Raised $Pco_2$ (when disease is well established)
*D*. Chest X-ray often shows chronic inflammatory changes
*E*. Diffusing capacity and *k*CO only mildly decreased with normal or slightly reduced total lung capacity
*F*. Often episodes of right-sided heart-failure

3. The *intermediate* or *indeterminate* type (Type X) show in some cases a mixture of findings and cannot be definitely assigned to Type A or Type B and hence are called Type X. However, some Type X patients will show little in the way of physiological disorder other than their airways obstruction and these are probably simple milder variants of the 'bronchitic' type.

Table 3—Main distinguishing features in patients with chronic airways obstruction

| | Chronic bronchitis | Emphysema | Asthma |
|---|---|---|---|
| Airways obstruction | Reversible or irreversible | Irreversible | Reversible |
| Total lung capacity | Normal or slightly reduced | Markedly increased | Normal (may be raised in acute attack) |
| Diffusing capacity | Normal or slightly decreased | Markedly decreased | Normal |
| Arterial oxygen tension | Reduced | Reduced (slightly) | Reduced in acute attack |
| Arterial $CO_2$ tension | Normal or raised | Normal or low | Normal or low |
| Chest X-ray | Normal or inflammatory changes. Later cardiac enlargement | Normal or areas of deficient vascularity | Normal (may show 'over-inflation' in acute attack) |
| Allergy | Not usual | Not present | Often present |
| Sex | Twice as common in males | Males only | Equal ratio |

The main aetiological factor in chronic bronchitis is, of course, cigarette smoking, although air pollution from internal combustion engines and domestic and industrial fuels play some part. In addition, there may be a genetic factor in that the condition is commonest in unskilled manual workers with a falling gradient through the social classes to the lowest incidence among professional and executive workers, but this could be explained also on environmental grounds. Infection also plays a prominent role in chronic bronchitis, if not in its initiation at least in the progress of the disease. A vicious cycle is established since excessive mucus predisposes to infection, and infection further irritates the mucosa.

The aetiology of emphysema is more obscure. It may be that it is initiated by infection or irritation (as yet unidentified), for some patients clearly date the onset to a respiratory infection or to being exposed to fog (especially 'smog'). On the other hand, it may be that the condition was already present but became noticed or exacerbated after such an episode. There is no doubt that localized or unilateral emphysema may develop as the sequel of respiratory infection in children, as has been clearly demonstrated by Reid (1967). The possibility of a genetic factor must also be considered. There is some evidence that some cases of emphysema, often of familial incidence, may be associated with deficiency of alpha-antitrypsin. This seems to be so in cases of basal emphysema. A possible explanation is that the enzyme deficiency permits an increase in circulating pancreatic trypsin which then has a destructive effect on the lung. If this is the mechanism then it might be expected that the bases fare worst since they are proportionately better perfused than the mid-zones and the upper zones.

The mortality from chronic bronchitis is high, around 90 deaths per 100,000 for men and around 30 per 100,000 for women, and involves mainly those over 50 years of age. Asthma accounts for about 4 deaths per

100,000 with a slightly higher mortality-rate in women than in men. The death-rate from asthma increases steeply with age which is probably why it appears to be uncommon in the elderly. In a personal series of 500 consecutive admissions for respiratory disease in patients over 65 years of age, only 8 (1·6 per cent) had uncomplicated asthma. Nevertheless, there are undoubted cases of late-onset asthma in the elderly with typical features of episodic wheezing dyspnoea, sputum and/or blood eosinophilia and raised serum IgE levels.

The management of chronic airways obstruction both during acute exacerbations and during the 'steady state' of remissions follows the same general principles with simply a different emphasis on the intensity of their application under given circumstances. These principles stem from the already discussed aetiological and pathophysiological features of the disease processes (*Fig.* 1).

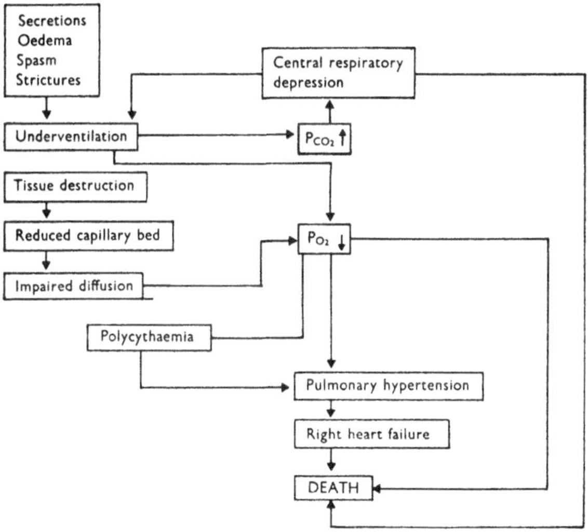


*Fig.* 1.—Some important factors in the pathogenesis of death from chronic airways obstruction.

## 1. SMOKING

Obviously cigarette smoking should be discouraged. This is extremely difficult for many patients, and in the elderly individuals it would often be inhumane to try to insist on complete abstinence.

## 2. AIR POLLUTION

This cannot in general be attacked directly by the physician, but patients should be advised to avoid fog. Fortunately the variety termed 'smog' which is particularly lethal is becoming rarer as the result of various clear-air programmes and automobile anti-pollution measures.

## 3. INFECTION

### A. Chronic

In general there are two important pathogens in chronic bronchitis: *Haemophilus influenzae* and *Streptococcus pneumoniae*.

For the treatment of chronic persistent infection, manifest by persistently purulent sputum, it is rational to attempt long-term antimicrobial therapy. In other patients with recurrent exacerbations it is just as effective to give an intermittent course of 4–10 days' duration as required. There are two equally effective antimicrobials available for this treatment—ampicillin and co-trimexazole. Tetracyclines are usually best avoided in the elderly because of side-effects and especially because of the risk of precipitating renal failure.

### B. Acute-on-Chronic

The treatment of mild exacerbations has already been described. More severe exacerbations warrant a higher dosage of antibiotic, e.g., ampicillin 1 g. 6-hourly. In very severe infections, or where there is doubt about absorption, intramuscular or even intravenous administration may be required.

Occasionally organisms other than *H. influenzae* or *Str. pneumoniae* may be responsible for the infection. If there is a possibility of resistant staphylococcal infection in the very ill patient it is logical to use a combination of ampicillin and flucloxacillin while waiting for the laboratory report.

*Klebsiella pneumoniae* is sometimes the underlying pathogen. My experience is that the laboratory reports of sensitivity tests for this organism are so misleading as to be useless. *In vivo* the organism seems only to respond to combined therapy with streptomycin and sulphonamide (or co-trimexazole).

A few seriously ill patients are found to have an infection due to *Pseudomonas pyocyanea* which is often difficult to deal with. Carbencillin will usually be required, and in life-threatening infection it may have to be given in large doses intravenously together with probenicid to raise the blood level and possibly concurrent intramuscular gentamycin.

*Bacillus proteus* sometimes poses a similar problem, though it is not always clear whether it is a true pathogen, and is treated with carbencillin. Reports of *Escherichia coli* should generally be ignored for in most cases it is a contaminant.

## 4. BRONCHOSPASM

The effective bronchodilators fall into three groups: β-adrenergic stimulators, xanthines and corticosteroid (including corticotrophins). Anti-cholinergics and antihistamines are not clinically useful.

### A. β-adrenergic Stimulators

The newer drugs in this group are relatively selective β-2 stimulators and have largely replaced the older sympathomimetics. The major importance of this in the elderly is that the new drugs have little or no effect on the heart and bladder. The two drugs of this type which are readily available are salbutamol and terbutaline between which there is little to choose. Both are administered in aerosol or tablet form, but, in addition, terbutaline is available for subcutaneous injection.

One potential hazard which has not yet been eliminated is that in some patients aerosol administration may increase the hypoxaemia already present. This is not usually of clinical importance except in status asthmaticus when overdosage may cause death. In the ambulant patient this increased hypoxaemia does not seem to occur during exercise, and in hospital an ill patient would almost certainly be given oxygen as well.

**B. Xanthines**

There is a wide variety of choice in this group, mainly in order to try to eliminate the chief side-effect, i.e., nausea. In general it may be said that the neutral theophylline derivatives are best tolerated, e.g., proxphylline. They may be administered intraveneously, orally, rectally or intramuscularly. The intravenous route is very useful in acute situations, the rectal route permits a sustained effect (about 6 hours); but there is some doubt about the efficiency of oral and intramuscular administration. Apart from the major side-effect of gastric irritation, they may produce tachycardia.

**C. Corticosteroids**

In certain circumstances corticosteroids (or corticotrophins) may be the most potent bronchodilators of all. The indications for their use are:

i. Status asthmaticus, which by definition implies failure of response to the usual bronchodilators. Here, unless there are clear contra-indications, the use of steroids is mandatory.

ii. Overwhelming infection, as a non-specific supporting measure until other therapy takes effect.

iii. Chronic obstruction not responsive to other bronchodilators. Obstruction cannot be labelled 'irreversible' until adequate corticosteroid therapy has been tried.

In the acute stages it is usual to give an initial dose of intravenous hydrocortisone and to commence oral corticosteroid dosage at the same time. This may only be needed for 1 or 2 weeks.

In long-term treatment it is essential to reduce steroid dosage to the minimum offering adequate symptomatic relief.

It is often possible to achieve a small mean daily dosage by using intramuscular triamcinolone acetonide at intervals of 3–6 weeks. More recently it has become possible to achieve satisfactory relief with an aerosol preparation of beclomethasone, with a much smaller average daily dosage.

Age is no barrier to the use of corticosteroids, but the elderly are more likely to suffer side-effects and a careful follow-up is necessary.

It is desirable that some objective measure should be used in assessing the response to bronchodilator therapy. The best measure is the percentage increase in $FEV_1$ over the base-line level (more than 20 per cent being a significant response), i.e.,

$$\frac{FEV_1 \text{after bronchodilator} - FEV_1 \text{before bronchodilator}}{FEV_1 \text{ before bronchodilator}}.$$

Alternatively, the peak flow-rate can be used with a similar calculation of response. It is particularly important to be able to demonstrate a worth-while response to corticosteroids in view of the potential hazards.

## 5. MUCOSAL OEDEMA

It is probable that some of the 'bronchodilator' action of corticosteroids is the result of reduction of inflammatory oedema. Similarly, aerosol sympathomimetics may exert a shrinking action on bronchial mucosa. Oedema will of course resolve as infection comes under control with antimicrobials. In some cases removal from offending allergens will help, and in others the administration of sodium cromoglycate may, by blocking allergic reactions, prevent oedema from occurring. The administration of sodium cromoglycate by a special insufflator aerosol may be dramatically helpful in the true asthmatic and some chronic bronchitics with asthma.

## 6. SECRETIONS

The expectoration of secretions is a natural protective mechanism and is to be encouraged. As a general rule, therefore, suppression of coughing is not recommended unless there is a dry irritating cough. Theoretically a preparation which reduced the frequency of coughing without rendering expectoration less effective would be of value but, despite claims to the contrary, it is doubtful whether such a preparation exists.

*Postural drainage* with or without percussion is probably the most useful measure in clearing the bronchi. The problem is that many elderly patients just will not tolerate being tipped, in which position respiration may become more difficult or cardiac embarrassment may occur or severe headache may develop.

*Sputum viscosity* tends to depend to some extent on the state of general hydration. Ensuring an adequate fluid intake may solve the immediate problem in some patients. This may, however, be difficult if faced with a patient in cardiac failure. Of the many attempts made to reduce sputum viscosity by the use of a variety of agents, none are as successful as inhalation of warm micro-aerosolized water. There is little (if any) convincing evidence of the effectiveness of enzymes, cysteine derivatives, detergents, iodine preparations or bromhexine as 'mucolytics'. Similarly there is no convincing evidence that substances such as guiac or ipecachuana are effective expectorants.

Bronchoscopy with aspiration, or even tracheostomy, may be required in acutely ill patients when the simpler measures have failed. This should not be undertaken unless the patient was reasonably well and definitely mobile prior to the current illness, otherwise one is merely prolonging an unpleasant and distressing state, delaying the inevitable conclusion without producing any worth-while benefit.

## 7. UNDERVENTILATION

Alveolar underventilation is present in a greater or lesser degree in all patients with chronic airways obstruction. This leads to hypoxaemia with or without carbon dioxide retention.

Measures to relieve bronchial obstruction may suffice to increase ventilation but if a dangerous degree of hypoxaemia ($Po_2$ less than 40 mm. Hg) persists or if the carbon dioxide tension is high ($Pco_2$ more than 65 mm. Hg) and especially if $CO_2$ tension is rising rapidly, other measures may be required.

The role of respiratory stimulants in the management of this situation is still subject to dispute. Some authors state didactically that they have no value. Others put forward a theoretical argument that conceivably the increased work of the respiratory muscles produced may use more oxygen than the increase in oxygen uptake produced by the stimulant. My own view, shared by others, is that there is a definite place for the use of these agents and I have no doubt in my own mind that many patients have been dramatically improved or spared assisted ventilation by their timely administration.

A number of drugs have been proposed as respiratory stimulants. Two which appear to have stood the test of time are prethcamide and amiphenazole, both of which may be given intravenously or intramuscularly, but, for reasons which are not understood, prethcamide seems more effective intramuscularly while amiphenazole seems more effective intravenously. Ethamivan and doxopram may also be effective intravenously.

The use of oral respiratory stimulants in the long-term treatment of patients with chronic underventilation has not been supported with any convincing evidence.

A steady rise in $CO_2$ tension will, if uncorrected, eventually lead to death. Under such conditions the question of assisted ventilation must be considered. Fortunately, in practice, this decision does not often have to be faced especially since the advent of controlled oxygen administration. Tracheostomy with assisted ventilation is seldom justified in the elderly unless the patient was previously able to fend for himself. In the very old it can only be justified in the case of an 'Einstein' or a 'Picasso'! I do not believe that it is right to create 'vegetables' and then squander valuable resources in maintaining them. If, however, there is real prospect of a return to fully independent existence then age should be no barrier.

It has already been stated that hypoxaemia is a feature of underventilation, and clearly oxygen administration is required in acute exacerbations when hypoxaemia can reach danger level. The problem with oxygen therapy in the past was that giving 100 per cent oxygen in these patients may depress respiration thus leading to further $CO_2$ retention and death. The mechanism of this is that many of these patients have become unresponsive to changes of $CO_2$ tension (the normal stimulus to respiration) and instead depend on hypoxaemia for their respiratory drive. The administration of oxygen will relieve their hypoxaemia but destroy their respiratory stimulus. To overcome this problem, there are now available masks for delivering oxygen-enriched air (controlled oxygen therapy). Thus there are Ventimasks delivering 24 or 28 per cent oxygen, the Edinburgh and the MC non-rebreathing masks delivering 25–30 per cent oxygen and the Hafoe head tent with settings for 24, 28 and 32 per cent oxygen. In the occasional patient who will tolerate neither mask nor head tent, oxygen enrichment of inspired air may be obtained by using nasal catheter spectacles with the rate of delivery being not more than 1 litre per min.

In a few patients even the slight oxygen enrichment provided by a 24 per cent mask may be sufficient to depress respiration to the extent of causing a rise in $CO_2$ tension. It is particularly in such patients that respiratory stimulants are useful.

The use of oxygen as long-term therapy has mostly been limited to the 'emphysematous' type of patients. Some of these patients are able to improve their exercise tolerance with the aid of a light-weight portable re-chargeable oxygen cylinder. It may be determined by trial and error whether this helps an individual patient. As a generalization it may be said that if maximum exercise is doubled by this method then it is likely to be of value to the patient in his daily life.

## 8. RIGHT-SIDED HEART FAILURE (COR PULMONALE)

The first line of treatment in established right heart failure is the administration of diuretic therapy. Depending on severity and response this may vary from a thiazide (with potassium supplement) on alternate days to a combination of frusemide or ethacrynic acid with amiloride and/or spironolactone and/or triamterine, in large daily doses. If massive doses are required it is essential to keep close check on electrolyte levels in the blood and to reduce to smaller maintenance doses as soon as possible.

The place of digitalis is still controversial. Obviously if there is rapid atrial fibrillation there is no argument. My own practice is not to use digitalis unless there is inadequate response to diuretic therapy. The preparations most suitable for use in the elderly are digoxin 0·0625 mg. tablets and lanatoside-C 0·25 mg. tablets. The main hazard is that digitalis itself may produce an arrythmia, especially if serum potassium is low (which it may well be as the result of diuretic therapy).

Strict fluid and salt restriction are not usually necessary but moderation is advised.

*Chapter Six*

# Bronchial Carcinoma

THE peak mortality of bronchial carcinoma in males has been steadily rising to the higher age-groups, with the peak now in the over 70-year group. The incidence on females is rising in all age-groups.

The relationship with cigarette smoking is well known, but in addition certain occupations carry a lung-cancer risk through exposure to chemicals such as chromate, nickel, arsenic or to mineral fibres such as asbestos.

Histologically, just over half of the cases of bronchial carcinoma are squamous celled, just under a half are anaplastic (including oat-celled) and the remainder are adenocarcinoma and alveolar-cell carcinoma (basal-cell carcinoma).

## PRESENTATION

1. Asymptomatic routine chest X-ray
2. Respiratory symptoms: recent cough, sputum, dyspnoea, haemoptysis or increased severity of such symptoms
3. General ill health; weight-loss (not an early feature)
4. Metastatic effects—especially cerebral
5. Complications, e.g. pneumonia, effusion, neuropathy
6. Pain—bony or pleuritic

## COMMON PHYSICAL FINDINGS

1. Finger clubbing
2. Atelectasis
3. Pneumonia
4. Pleural effusion
5. Localized tenderness
6. Hard enlarged lymph-nodes, especially supraclavicular
7. Liver nodules
8. 'Pancoast' syndrome (high apical tumour)
   *A.* Brachial neuralgia (C8, T1, T2 roots)
   *B.* Horner's syndrome (cervical sympathetic)
   *C.* Hoarseness (recurrent laryngeal)

## IMPORTANT X-RAY FINDINGS

1. Unilateral hilar enlargement
2. Peripheral shadows—nodule, mass, irregular opacities (both homogeneous and non-homogeneous), irregular cavitation
3. Collapse or consolidation (distal to neoplasm)
4. Pleural effusion
5. Mediastinal enlargment
6. Elevation of hemi-diaphragm (paralysis confirmed by fluoroscopy)
7. Rib erosion
8. Lymphangitic carcinomatosis (bilateral hilar enlargment with streaky shadows fanning out into the lungs)
9. Pericardial effusion

## COMPLICATIONS

**1. Mechanical**

*A.* Atelectasis
*B.* Superior vena caval obstruction

**2. Inflammatory**

*A*. Pneumonia
*B*. Abscess

**3. Pleural**

*A*. Effusion (often blood-stained)—recurs rapidly after aspiration and may contain malignant cells.
*B*. Malignant infiltration

**4. Cardiac**

*A*. Malignant infiltration of myocardium
*B*. Malignant infiltration of pericardium

**5. Metastatic**

*A*. May be anywhere
*B*. Particularly prone to occur in: cervical and mediastinal lymph-nodes, liver, bones and brain

**6. Neurological**

*A*. Phrenic paralysis
*B*. Recurrent laryngeal paralysis
*C*. Brachial plexus invasion
*D*. Brain (often simulates primary tumour)
*E*. Neuropathies
  i. Sensory
  ii. Motor
  iii. Cerebellar degeneration
  iv. Peripheral neuropathy
  v. Dementia
  vi. Myopathy
  vii. Dermatomyositis

These neuropathies may precede or follow the primary neoplasm and may fluctuate (even to full remission) independently.

**7. Endocrine**

*A.* Hyponatraemia
*B.* Hypercorticosteroidism ('Cushingoid')
*C.* Hypercalcaemia
*D.* Carcinoid
*E.* Hyperthyroidism
*F.* Hypoglycaemia
*G.* Red-cell aplasia
*H.* Adrenal failure (metastases)

**8. Hypertrophic Pulmonary Osteoarthropathy**

## DIAGNOSIS

1. X-ray (as previously described)—including tomograms
2. Sputum cytology—often very helpful
3. Pleural biopsy and fluid cytology
4. Bronchoscopy—seldom indicated in the over-70 age-group as most surgeons will not operate (but *see below* under treatment)—under 70 worth while if no contra-indications to eventual surgery (otherwise a purely academic exercise)
5. Bronchography—same criteria as for bronchoscopy; may demonstrate bronchial block beyond reach of bronchoscope
6. Barium swallow may demonstrate mediastinal lymph-node enlargement or oesophageal involvement
7. Lung scanning may show vascular deficiency distal to suspicious lesion.

## DIFFERENTIAL DIAGNOSIS

1. Main lesions to be differentiated are:
   *A.* Tuberculosis
   *B.* Lung abscess (non-malignant)

   C. Pneumonia (not distal to an obstruction)
   D. Benign tumour (fairly rare)
   E. Pulmonary infarct
2. Slow resolution of 'pneumonia' (i.e., more than 6 weeks in the elderly) suggests:
   A. Carcinoma
   B. Tuberculosis
   C. Pulmonary infarct
3. Other causes of pleural effusion (q.v.)
4. Other causes of round peripheral shadow on X-ray:
   A. Well-defined hair-line margin against diagnosis carcinoma
   B. Small satellite shadows favour tuberculosis
   C. Linear radiations favour carcinoma

## TREATMENT

The general outlook is poor. The survival rate for all cases is about 1 per cent at the end of 3 years after diagnosis, and this figure includes those which were actually resectable.

### 1. Surgery

Many surgeons will not operate on patients more than 70 years of age. Some surgeons who do operate regardless of age find that a small proportion of the total are resectable, and of these about 30 per cent survive for 4 years. The question is whether the patients have had 4 more worth-while years of life and this is debatable.

Even over the age of 60 the operative mortality is twice that of younger patients and some patients survive for 5 years without therapy. One of the major problems in medical practice is how to apply group statistics (in this case, concerning prognosis) to the individual patient. The only advice I can give is that each case must be considered on its own merits.

Quite apart from these considerations there are a number of definite contra-indications to surgery:

*A.* Respiratory infection
*B.* Pulmonary embolism
*C.* Metastases
*D.* $FEV_1$ less than 40 per cent of predicted or $CO_2$ retention
*E.* Persistent pleural effusion
*F.* Neoplasm close to left main bronchus
*G.* Brachial plexus invasion
*H.* Other serious disease

## 2. Radiotherapy

This has a place in palliation:

*A.* Mediastinal compression (superior vena caval) is often relieved for a while.
*B.* Haemoptyses are often stopped for a while.
*C.* Pain is sometimes relieved for a while.
*D.* Bronchial obstruction may sometimes be relieved (and sometimes be made worse).
*E.* Occasionally cough is temporarily relieved.

## 3. Cytotoxic Therapy

The same considerations apply as to radiotherapy. In addition intrapleural instillation may delay recurrence of effusion.

The main drugs used are mustine hydrochloride and cyclophosphamide. Both may be given intravenously (divided doses may be given but total dose infusion is better) and both produce marrow depression. Cyclophosphamide has the disadvantage of producing alopecia, but has the doubtful advantage of being able to be given orally for long-term treatment. The only real justification for the latter is for relief of bone pain.

The potential for treatment is indeed bleak. All that can generally be offered is relief of pain and of distressing cough. Electrical cordotomy is sometimes successful in the relief of pain, but carries the hazard of producing a hemiparesis. Various analgesics will inevitably be tried in the hope of avoiding narcotics, but usually a time comes when it is necessary to use them to produce adequate pain amelioration. Irritating cough may be controlled by codeine or similar drugs but the most effective is diamorphine (heroin). This is, of course, a highly effective analgesic also and when the time comes there should be no hesitation over using it.

*Chapter Seven*

# The Pneumonias

ANATOMICALLY pneumonias may be lobar, segmental or lobular (bronchopneumonic) in type. Most pneumonias are infections although it is not always possible to isolate the organism responsible, especially in the elderly debilitated bronchitic patient. Often there is failure to isolate the organism because of previous antimicrobial therapy. The main organisms found in the pneumonias are—*Streptococcus pneumoniae*, *Staphylococcus pyogenes*, *Klebsiella pneumonia* and *Mycobacterium tuberculosis*.

The mortality-rate, not unexpectedly, rises with age (greater in males than in females), but 'pneumonia' is often a terminal event in some other illness or used as a convenient label on the death certificate.

The functional result of consolidation is to produce a 'shunt' effect (i.e., circulation continues through unaerated lung tissue) which produces arterial hypoxaemia. Bronchopneumonia commonly occurs in bronchitic subjects resulting in increase in hypoxaemia together with hypercapnia.

## PREDISPOSING FACTORS

1. Exposure to cold—often associated with hypothermia
2. Following operations—poor cough reflex, weak musculature

3. Following common cold—especially bronchitic subjects
4. Distal to bronchial obstruction
5. Secondary to alcoholism (which is usually occult in the elderly)
6. Extreme age (decrease in body's defences)

## CLINICAL FEATURES

### 1. Lobar Pneumonia

*A.* PNEUMOCOCCAL

Flushed appearance, cyanosis, tachypnoea, labial herpes, pyrexia (but not always in elderly), diminished chest movement, pleuritic pain, dullness, increased vocal resonance, pleural rub, bronchial breathing and whispering pectoriloquoy

X-ray appearance: hazy uniform shadow corresponding to anatomical lobe (but not always whole lobe). Polymorph leucocytosis (but not always in elderly). Raised erythrocyte sedimentation rate (if still raised after 6 weeks consider myelomatosis, collagenosis, carcinoma)

*B.* STAPHYLOCOCCAL

Often very severe; mostly associated with influenza epidemics. X-ray frequently shows abscess formation (small, multiple)

*C.* TUBERCULOUS

Failure to respond to usual antimicrobials; positive sputum test

*D.* KLEBSIELLA

Tendency to abscess and empyema formation; frequently involves upper lobes; high mortality in elderly males

**2. Segmental Pneumonias**

Generally due to mechanical factors, e.g., aspiration and often are mild with virtually chest X-ray changes only. These cases behave like lobar pneumonias.

**3. Bronchopneumonias**

Characteristic X-ray appearance is of patchy shadows (which may be unilateral); often associated with chronic bronchitis; may be viral (especially influenzal), or due to infection with *Haemophilus influenzae*, *Str. pneumoniae* or *Staph. pyogenes*. Hypostatic pneumonia in elderly bed-ridden patients is due to invasion of retained secretions and oedema. Fever is usually present (but not necessarily in elderly) with cough and purulent sputum (but this may not be expectorated). There may be fine crackles and patchy bronchial breathing; occasionally a pleural rub may be heard; there are often cyanosis and confusion due to hypoxaemia; there may be tremor and coma due to $CO_2$ retention; in some cases there may be gross bubbling sounds and patient may drown in his own secretions; right-heart failure is frequently precipitated by bronchopneumonia.

## DIFFERENTIAL DIAGNOSIS

**1. Pulmonary Infarction**

Sudden onset, non-purulent sputum, deep venous thrombosis (this may only appear later; ultrasound or radiofibrinogen tests useful), repeated episodes of pleurisy, fresh shadowing on X-ray during antimicrobial therapy or failure to respond should arouse suspicion.

**2. Tuberculous Pleural Effusion**

Lymphocytic fluid, absence of polymorph leucocytosis, and positive pleural biopsy are the hallmarks of tuberculous pleural effusion.

**3. Carcinoma**

Persistence of shadowing more than 6 weeks despite antimicrobial therapy is very suspicious; hilar enlargement.

**4. Severe Chronic Bronchitis**

Absence of bronchopneumonic shadowing on X-ray is the main distinguishing feature.

**5. Other Segmental Lesions**

Carcinoma, infarcts (especially if multiple) or tuberculous lesions may produce segmented shadowing on X-ray.

## PREVENTION

Wherever possible poor ventilation should be remedied, overcrowding avoided, atmospheric pollution reduced, cigarette smoking stopped, alcohol withdrawn and cold avoided.

In the chronic bronchitic antimicrobial therapy should be given promptly for any infection, even of the upper respiratory tract, together with postural coughing (when tolerated).

## TREATMENT

**1. General**

Give attention to comfort, hydration, provision of commode, leg exercises.

**2. Relief of Pleurisy**

*Non-bronchitic* may have 10 mg. morphine (or equivalent of other similar drug).

*Bronchitic* must not be given narcotic (except that if pain is not relieved by other analgesics such as paracetamol, dextropropoxyphene, dihydrocodeine or pantazocine) pethidine may be used together with the analeptic levallorphan (which counteracts the respiratory depression).

### 3. Oxygen

Oxygen should be given if any cyanosis (24–28 per cent for the bronchitic).

### 4. Postural Drainage

This, with or without percussion of the chest, will aid expectoration.

### 5. Antimicrobial Therapy

*A*. At home (usually the mild case) the choice usually lies between penicillin, ampicillin, co-trimexazole or a tetracycline (however, most tetracyclines may precipitate renal failure in the elderly; it is claimed that doxycycline does not have this drawback).

*B*. In hospital the moderate case can usually afford to wait at least for the Gram-stained smear, if not for sensitivity reports. While waiting, one of above antimicrobials can be started and changed later if necessary.

*C*. In hospital the severe case is best treated with combined antimicrobials from the start, adjusting as required when sensitivity tests are reported. Ampicillin plus flucloxacillin gives good cover.

*D*. In hospital the desperately ill case should be given streptomycin plus penicillin plus flucloxacillin plus corticosteroids in the first instance.

## COMPLICATIONS

1. Pleural effusion (common)
2. Empyema (rare)
3. Lung abscess—with staphylococcal or *Klebsiella* infection

4. Spontaneous pneumothorax—with staphylococcal infection
5. Peripheral thrombophlebitis
6. Circulatory failure

## PROGNOSIS

Mortality increases with age, bronchitis and complicating or coincident disease. The mortality rate in the elderly is around 10 per cent.

## SEQUELAE

1. Resolution may leave residual fibrosis.
2. Recurrence at the same site may occur—neoplasm or bronchiectasis.
3. Recurrent attacks at different sites—infarcts, myelomatosis or aspiration.
4. Lipoid pneumonia may occur in elderly persons who use oily nose drops or aperients. It produces a diffuse interstitial pneumonia which clinically often manifests as cough, sputum and dyspnoea. Chest X-ray shows small nodules, or basal interstitial fibrosis, or multiple reticular shadows.

*Chapter Eight*

# Pulmonary Tuberculosis

## MILIARY TUBERCULOSIS

### Pathogenesis

Recrudescence of old primary focus discharging infective material into the circulation. Now more common in the elderly than in the young.

### Predisposing Factors

1. Corticosteroid therapy
2. Leukaemias
3. Other debilitating diseases, e.g., diabetes mellitus

### Pathology

Small foci in lungs; may be similar foci in spleen, liver, kidneys, serous sacs (producing effusions); rarely 'malignant' septicaemia; bone marrow may be involved.

### Clinical Findings

1. Meningitis
2. Fever (many present as pyrexia of undetermined origin (PUO))
3. Malaise and loss of weight
4. Often no chest signs until very late (diffuse crackles)
5. Spleen occasionally palpable
6. Choroidal tubercles rare in adults

**Chest X-ray**

1. May be *normal!*
2. Evenly distributed 1–2 mm. shadows (miliary) are present.
3. Bilateral pleural effusions may occur.

**Diagnosis**

1. Classical picture comprises fever, enlarged spleen, choroidal tubercles and miliary shadowing on X-ray: not often seen.

2. Tuberculin test not very helpful:
   *A.* May be negative (or weakly positive) in any elderly subject.
   *B.* May be negative in presence of severe infection.
   *C.* May be positive from past infection anyway.

3. Biopsy—liver, bone marrow, pleura may provide positive evidence.

4. Therapeutic test with antituberculous drugs is advised whenever there is any suspicion of this diagnosis (the best combination is probably rifampicin plus ethambutol plus isoniazid; if streptomycin is used in a therapeutic test one is always left with the unanswerable question: 'Could this have been due to an occult coccal infection which has responded to streptomycin?').

**Prognosis**

1. Untreated—fatal

2. Treated (especially if early diagnosis)—good; probably no sequelae.

**Complications**

1. Pleural effusion (may have to be differentiated from SLE).

2. Hypokalaemia—may even require intravenous replacement if patient is very ill.

3. Blood dyscrasias—many described, including aplastic anaemia, pancytopenia, leucopenia, agranulocytosis,

leukaemoid pattern, leuco-erythroblastic anaemia, purpura and polycythaemia vera. Most respond as miliary responds to antituberculous therapy.

**Treatment**

1. Antituberculous drugs: rifampicin, ethambutol, isoniazid.

2. Corticosteroids may be needed for desperately ill patients—can usually be discontinued after few weeks.

## POST-PRIMARY PULMONARY TUBERCULOSIS

**Pathogenesis**

Rapidly becoming a disease of the elderly. Occurs as reactivation of primary focus acquired in childhood, or of a post-primary lesion which had previously been contained by the host's defences.

**Pathology**

The characteristic lesion is caseation surrounded by Langhan's giant cells. Liquefaction of caseous tissue and its evacuation via the bronchial tree leads to cavity formation. Tuberculous pneumonia, pulmonary fibrosis and calcification may occur.

**Functional Abnormalities**

1. Restrictive
   - *A.* Pleural thickening
   - *B.* Pulmonary fibrosis
2. Obstructive
   - *A.* Compensatory emphysema
   - *B.* Coincidental bronchitis
   - *C.* Bronchostenosis
3. Loss of functional tissue may produce impaired diffusion.

4. Pulmonary hypertension (leading to right-heart failure) may occur eventually as a result of severe extensive lung destruction.

**Symptoms**

1. None—lesion seen on X-ray
2. General (non-specific)
   *A*. Tiredness
   *B*. Malaise
   *C*. Weight-loss
   *D*. Fever
   *E*. Difficulty in concentrating
   *F*. Anorexia
   *G*. Dyspepsia
3. Respiratory
   *A*. Cough
   *B*. Sputum
   *C*. Haemoptysis
   *D*. Chest pain (pleurisy, dull ache or cough fracture)
   *E*. Dyspnoea
   *F*. Localized wheeze (bronchostenosis)
   *G*. Pneumonia
   *H*. Recurrent 'colds' anteceding tuberculosis

**Physical Signs**

1. Often none of any significance
2. May be
   *A*. Post-tussive crackles in upper zones
   *B*. Signs of consolidation
   *C*. Localized wheeze
   *D*. Tracheal deviation

**Chest X-ray**

This is *very* important; a normal film virtually excludes tuberculosis except that a very small lesion may escape notice (observer error); a very rare condition which does not show X-ray changes is tuberculous bronchitis *per se.* Some of the possible changes have been discussed in Chapter Four. Fuller discussion is outside the scope of this book.

**Sputum**

This too is *very* important. Sputum should be examined as smear (Ziehl-Neelsen) and cultured. Culture results usually take 8 weeks before being considered negative. Guinea-pig inoculation has now been virtually abandoned since a series of cultures gives an equally high yield of positive results. If sputum cannot be obtained, gastric washings or laryngeal swabs should be examined and cultured.

**Other Laboratory Tests**

1. White cell count usually normal or decreased; not of much significance.
2. Erythrocyte sedimentation rate often raised; not of diagnostic value; of doubtful value in follow-up.
3. Anaemia common—usually normocytic and improved *parri passu* with the tuberculosis; there may be iron deficiency; there may occasionally be a macrocytic anaemia.
4. Liver function not infrequently abnormal even before administering any drugs; usually improves as tuberculosis improves.

**Tuberculin Test**

For reasons given under 'Miliary tuberculosis' (p. 73), this test is not really worth doing in the elderly.

**Signs of Activity**

1. Positive sputum
2. Cough, tiredness, loss of weight
3. Persistent crackles

4. X-ray:
   *A.* Cavitation (unless already treated)
   *B.* 'Soft' shadows
   *C.* Extensive shadows
   *D.* Extending shadows

**Differential Diagnosis**

1. PNEUMONIA

Pneumonia persisting longer than 3 weeks despite adequate antibiotic therapy is unlikely to be pyogenic; persisting after 6 weeks is unlikely to be viral.

2. BRONCHIAL CARCINOMA

Hilar enlargement is suspicious; tuberculosis and carcinoma may coexist; satellite lesions and calcification in favour of tuberculosis (tomograms may be needed); sputum examination for malignant cells as well as for tubercle bacilli should be undertaken.

3. LUNG ABSCESS

Patient more likely to be ill, leucocytosis more likely; staphylococci, *Klebsiella* or actinomycosis organisms.

4. PNEUMOCONIOSIS

Complicated by added tuberculosis: X-ray may not be diagnostic; sputum examination required.

5. PULMONARY INFARCTION

Presence of predisposing factors, especially deep venous thrombosis (*see* Chapter Nine).

**Complications**

1. Pleurisy with effusion
2. Empyema (may be encysted)
3. Laryngitis
4. Right ventricular failure
5. Amyloidosis

6. Mycetoma—infection of old cavity with *Aspergillus*
7. Carcinoma—may originate in old tuberculous scar
8. Hypokalaemia—not uncommon in elderly

**Treatment**

1. IF EVIDENCE OF ACTIVITY

2. WHERE DOUBTFUL OF ACTIVITY
   *A.* As a therapeutic trial
   *B.* While awaiting sputum results
   *C.* Where there is risk of contacts
   *D.* Where in doubt between carcinoma or tuberculosis

3. HOSPITAL ADMISSION ONLY IF
   *A.* Very ill
   *B.* Very extensive disease
   *C.* Direct positive sputum (smear)
   *D.* Social reasons

4. ANTITUBERCULOUS DRUGS
   *A.* Combination of two or more *always* required
   *B.* Best combination at present (particularly for elderly) is rifampicin plus ethambutol plus isoniazid for 3 months followed by rifampicin plus isoniazid or rifampicin plus ethambutol (depending on sensitivity results) for a further 3 months for small lesions or a further 6 months for larger lesions
   *C.* Dosage schedules:
      i. *Rifampicin*: 450 or 600 mg. (depending on weight) as single daily dose 30 min. before a meal
      ii. *Isoniazid*: 300 mg. daily—divided or single doses
      iii. *Ethambutol*: 15 mg. per kg. of body-weight per day—divided or single doses

*D*. Toxicity:

i. *Rifampicin*: occasional liver dysfunction (usually transient); tears and urine turn pink (of no significance)

ii. *Isoniazid*: non-toxic in dosage recommended

iii. *Ethambutol*: retrobulbar neuritis (very rare in dosage recommended)

*Chapter Nine*

# Pulmonary Thrombo-embolic Disease

## AETIOLOGY

PULMONARY emboli almost invariably arise from detachment of clots formed in ileofemoral or pelvic veins. Occasionally they may arise from the right ventricle following myocardial infarction of apex or septum. Parodoxical embolism is excessively rare. Thrombosis may occur *in situ* in congested lungs.

## PREDISPOSING FACTORS

1. Immobilization
   *A.* Following fractures
   *B.* Following cerebrovascular incidents
   *C.* Sitting for prolonged periods in the same position
   *D.* Prolonged bed-rest for any reason
2. Congestive cardiac failure
3. Malignant disease
4. Polycythaemia
5. Obesity
6. Increasing age: a common cause of death in the elderly
7. Trauma to legs or pelvis, including surgery
8. Varicose veins (although still a matter of dispute)
9. Steroids: particularly oestrogens, but also corticosteroids.

Sometimes no cause is found. Some emboli may be other than clots, i.e., fat, tumour cells, air or even foreign bodies.

## PATHOLOGY

Pulmonary infarction occurs only if medium or large branches of a pulmonary artery are blocked, and there is pre-existing pulmonary congestion, and the patient survives for at least 2 days. Organization of an infarct is not uncommon. Repeated emboli are the rule. Occasionally an infarct becomes infected and produces a lung abscess.

## CLINICAL EFFECTS

1. Pulmonary embolism may produce:
   *A*. Acute right-heart dilatation with dilatation of neck veins and engorgement of the liver
   *B*. Chronic right ventricular hypertrophy
   *C*. Myocardial necrosis with hypoxaemia and shock (reflex coronary insufficiency?)
   *D*. Bronchospasm (neurogenic reflex?)
   *E*. Pulmonary oedema
2. Massive embolization often produces:
   *A*. Straining at stool
   *B*. Shock
   *C*. Hypotension
   *D*. Tachycardia
   *E*. Tachypnoea
   *F*. ECG changes
3. Moderate embolization causing infarction may produce any combination of
   *A*. Cough
   *B*. Haemoptysis
   *C*. Pleurisy
   *D*. Jaundice (mild)

*E*. Anginal pain
*F*. Fever
*G*. Cardiac dysrhythmias
*H*. Dizziness or syncope
*I*. Nausea or vomiting
*J*. Precipitation of cardiac failure, intensification of pre-existing cardiac failure, refractoriness to treatment of pre-existing cardiac failure

4. Small emboli may produce
*A*. Tachypnoea
*B*. Tachycardia
*C*. Hypotension
*D*. Syncope
*E*. Exertional dyspnoea
*F*. Fatigue

## SPECIAL INVESTIGATIONS

### 1. Biochemical

*A*. Raised serum LDH, with normal SGOT, and slightly raised bilirubin is said to be characteristic; occurs in about 50 per cent of cases.

### 2. ECG Changes

*A*. Deep S lead 1, deep Q lead 3, plus T inversion in leads 3 and $V_1$ to $V_4$
*B*. Right-bundle branch block
*C*. Various dysrhythmias

### 3. X-ray Changes

*A*. Pleural effusion
*B*. Linear atelectases
*C*. Elevation of hemidiaphragm
*D*. Irregular, or round, or wedge-shaped (rare!) shadows
*E*. Repeated emboli produce cor pulmonale

**4. Lung Scanning**

*A.* Macroaggregates of human albumen labelled with technetium-99 usually used.

*B.* Areas of diminished vascularity correlate well with angiographic evidence of blockage (but other lesions may cause diminished vascularity, e.g., fibrosis, pneumonia, neoplasm).

**5. Pulmonary Angiography**

*A.* Provides definite evidence of site or sites of blocked arteries.

**6. Deep Venous Thrombosis**

*A.* CLINICAL

Pain, tenderness and swelling of limb; positive Homan's sign (alternatively, tenderness of instep).

*B.* PHLEBOGRAPHY

Will delineate site and extent of thrombosis.

*C.* ULTRASOUND PROBE (utilizing Doppler effect)

Value mainly in demonstrating patency of vessels to exclude block.

*D.* RADIOACTIVE FIBRINOGEN

To delineate block—correlates quite well with phlebography.

## DIAGNOSIS

1. A high index of suspicion should be maintained.

2. Diagnosis should be considered in any patient confined to bed who develops any of the following symptoms:

*A.* Shock

*B.* Syncope

*C*. Precordial oppression
*D*. Pleuritic pain
*E*. Dyspnoea
*F*. Tachypnoea
*G*. Cyanosis

3. Diagnosis should be considered as likely cause of following symptoms and signs in patients with congestive failure, or in second postoperative week, or after myocardial infarction:

*A*. Unexplained fever
*B*. Pleural effusion
*C*. Increasing tachycardia

4. Radiographic consolidation not clearing despite antimicrobial therapy suspicious of infarction (or neoplasm).

5. The so-called classical triad of cough, pleurisy and haemoptysis is actually uncommon.

6. The so-called classical wedge-shaped X-ray shadow is uncommon.

7. Signs of deep venous thrombosis may not present until after embolization has occurred (or may never be present clinically).

## DIFFERENTIAL DIAGNOSIS

1. Pneumonia: in which there will be lack of appropriate history, purulent sputum, lack of ECG changes and response to antimicrobial therapy.

2. Haemoptysis: may occur in patient on anticoagulant therapy following myocardial infarction.

3. Myocardial infarction: distinguished usually by history, ECG and enzymes (SGOT raised early, LDH raised late); sometimes distinction cannot be definite.

4. Pleural effusion: other causes may have to be distinguished by examination of fluid, pleural biopsy, etc. (*see* Chapter Ten).

5. Pleuritic pain: other causes usually distinguishable from X-rays.

6. Dyspnoea: other causes need exclusion (*see* Chapter Two).

## PROGNOSIS

1. Massive—10 per cent survival without surgery.

2. Medium and small—usually recur; often final massive embolism; may improve with anticoagulant therapy or fibrinolytic therapy.

## TREATMENT

### 1. Prophylactic

*A.* Avoid prolonged bed rest; encourage leg exercises; allow use of commode

*B.* Avoid dehydration

*C.* Anticoagulate if immobilization unavoidable

*D.* Recognize and treat deep venous thrombosis

### 2. Deep Venous Thrombosis

*A.* Anticoagulant therapy with careful control of prothrombin levels.

*B.* Fibrinolytic therapy with streptokinase infusion may be very successful, but is very expensive and requires special facilities for control.

*C.* An alternative form of 'fibrinolytic' therapy without appreciable side-effects is the combination of the antidiabetic drug phenformin (50 mg. of sustained-release preparation twice daily) and the anabolic steroid ethylestrenol (4 mg. twice daily); presumably other anabolic steroids would also be effective in the combination, which has been shown to decrease serum fibrinogen, lower plasma thrombin and reduce platelet adhesiveness.

**3. Massive Embolism**

*A.* Pain relief—morphine
*B.* Hypotension—pressor agents, e.g., metaraminol
*C.* Hypoxaemia—oxygen inhalation
*D.* Atrial fibrillation—digitalize
*E.* Anticoagulate
*F.* Streptokinase if facilities
*G.* General resuscitation
*H.* Rarely embelectomy with cardiac by-pass

**4. Smaller, Single or Recurrent Emboli**

*A.* As for deep venous thrombosis
*B.* If recurrence despite these measures ligation of or plication of inferior vena cava may be considered

*Chapter Ten*

# Pleural Effusion

## PATHOLOGY

ACCUMULATION of fluid in the pleural cavity may be due to transudation or exudation.

**1. Transudates**

*A.* Usually protein less than 3 g. per cent and specific gravity less than 1·015

*B.* Usual causes are—congestive cardiac failure, hypoproteinemia, constrictive pericarditis, myxoedema

**2. Exudates**

*A.* Usually protein greater than 3 g. per cent and specific gravity greater than 1·015

*B.* Usual causes are

- i. Pneumonias: neutrophilic effusion
- ii. Pulmonary infarcts: often eosinophilic effusion
- iii. Malignancies: bloody effusion, rapidly recurring, may contain malignant cells
- iv. Tuberculosis: lymphocytic effusion

## CLINICAL FINDINGS

1. History of pleuritic pain (which usually disappears as fluid accumulates)
2. Signs of effusion

   *A.* Restricted movement

   *B.* Stony dullness

*C.* Weak or absent breath sounds, vocal fremitus and vocal resonance (at upper level of dullness there may be bronchial breathing)

*D.* Mediastinal shift away from large effusion

## CHEST X-RAY

1. Characteristically a dense homogeneous shadow with a curved upper border.

2. To distinguish from pleural thickening it may be desirable to take a film in lateral recumbency (fluid will shift).

3. There may be evidence of associated pathology *ab initio* or only after aspiration of fluid.

## INVESTIGATION

### 1. Aspiration with Biopsy

*A.* Abram's needle renders this a fairly innocuous procedure.

*B.* Histology 40 per cent positive in malignancy, 80 per cent positive in tuberculosis.

*C.* Complications (uncommon if procedure carried out skilfully)

- i. Pulmonary oedema—from too rapid removal of fluid
- ii. Circulatory collapse—from production of high negative pressure (where lung is bound down by adhesions) thus interfering with venous return
- iii. Air embolism—from tearing visceral pleura or entering a vessel
- iv. 'Pleural shock' = vasovagal attack from stimulation of pleura

v. Haemorrhage—from rupture of intercostal vessel
vi. Hydropneumothorax—from puncturing lung
vii. Haemoptysis—from puncturing lung

## 2. Characteristics of Fluid

*A.* MACROSCOPIC

i. Straw-coloured or amber—exudate
ii. Pale and watery—transudate
iii. Bloody (bright red to dark brown)—malignancy, pulmonary infarction, trauma, occasionally tuberculosis
iv. Purulent—empyema
v. Milky—presence of chyle

*B.* PROTEIN AND SPECIFIC GRAVITY

Overlap between results renders tests of little practicality.

*C.* CYTOLOGY

Often difficult to be certain of malignancy of cells in fluid (may be false positives)

*D.* CHEMISTRY

i. Fat—confirms chylothorax
ii. Glucose less than 20 mg. per cent consistent with rheumatoid disease
iii. Raised amylase—effusion associated with pancreatitis

*E.* BACTERIOLOGY

i. Culture for pyogenic bacteria
ii. Smear and culture for tubercle bacilli
iii. Culture for fungi

## TREATMENT

**1. Basic Condition**

Treat basic condition, e.g., pneumonia, congestive heart failure.

**2. Malignant effusion**

*A.* Can only be palliative.

*B.* Generally try to prevent recurrence for as long as possible

i. Intrapleural nitrogen mustard and systemic corticosteroid

ii. Intrapleural radioactive material, e.g., gold (in practice no better than mustine)

*C.* In the special case of effusion secondary to hormone-sensitive breast cancer effusion may be controlled by oestrogens and/or androgens.

**3. Tuberculous effusion**

*A.* Now more common in elderly.

*B.* Bilateral effusion may be due to miliary tuberculosis.

*C.* Aspiration followed by 6 weeks' systemic corticosteroids together with rifampicin plus ethambutol plus isoniazid; subsequently continue rifampicin plus isoniazid up to 6–9 months.

*Chapter Eleven*

# Fungal Infection

## ASPERGILLOSIS

### 1. Bacteriology

*A.* Spores ubiquitous
*B.* Main pathogen is *Aspergillus fumigatus*
*C.* Other varieties may be pathogenic in individual cases, i.e., *Aspergillus niger*, *Aspergillus flavius*, *Aspergillus nidulans*

### 2. Types of bronchopulmonary aspergillosis

*A.* ALLERGIC

i. Pulmonary infiltrates with asthma
ii. Eosinophilia in blood (more than 500 per $mm.^3$) and sputum (more than 20 per cent of white cells)
iii. *A. fumigatus* cultured from sputum
iv. Immediate (type I) skin hypersensitivity
v. Positive precipitin test (serum) in 70–90 per cent (Type III hypersensitivity)
vi. Bronchial hypersensitivity test positive in 90–100 per cent

*B.* ASPERGILLOMA (MYCETOMA)

i. Invasion of pre-existing cavity—usually tuberculous but occasionally cysts, bronchiectasis, abscess, etc.

ii. Haemoptysis common; cachexia later
iii. X-ray shows dense opacity separated from cavity wall by a 'halo' of air
iv. Precipitins usually present in serum
v. Positive skin test suggests that allergy coexists

*C.* NECROTIC
Occurs in debilitated subjects

*D.* DISSEMINATED
Related to serious underlying disease, e.g., malignancy, leukaemia, reticulosis, or to certain therapies, e.g., corticosteroids, cytotoxics, antibiotics

*E.* EXTRINSIC ALLERGIC ALVEOLITIS
i. Cough, sputum, dyspnoea
ii. Coarse crackles in chest; finger clubbing common
iii. Restrictive spirometric pattern with impaired diffusion
iv. X-ray: widely distributed micronodular pattern progressing to fibrosis with honeycombing
v. May occur as acute, subacute or chronic illness

**3. Treatment**

*A.* Allergic: infiltrates clear with corticosteroid therapy, type I reactions blocked by sodium cromoglycate, antifungal agents may help (e.g., natamycin (Pimafucin) inhalations).

*B.* Mycetoma: no therapy of any proven value.

*C.* Necrotic or disseminated: intravenous amphotericin B should be tried as possibly life-saving despite hazards of this antibiotic.

*D.* Fibrosing alveolitis: an appreciable number of patients may benefit from corticosteroid therapy.

## CANDIDIASIS (MONILIASIS)

### Predisposing Factors

1. Local trauma
2. Endocrinopathies
   *A*. Diabetes mellitus
   *B*. Hypoadrenalism
   *C*. Hypoparathyroidism
   *D*. Pancreatitis
   *E*. Hypothyroidism
3. Malnutrition
4. Malabsorption
5. Blood dyscrasias
6. Malignancies

BRONCHOPULMONARY CANDIDIASIS

1. Rare despite above factors.

2. *Bronchial*—plaques similar to those seen in throat; cough with sputum culture *repeatedly* positive; normal chest X-ray.

3. *Pulmonary*—fever, cough, haemoptysis; chest X-ray shows patchy opacities.

### Diagnosis

Largely dependent on awareness of predisposing factors, plus a series of positive sputum cultures.

### Treatment

1. Nystatin by inhalation (and also by oral route as gut is usually involved as well).

2. If patient seriously ill intravenous amphotericin B may be required.

5

*Chapter Twelve*

# Some Less Common Diseases

## 1. BRONCHIECTASIS

BRONCHIECTASIS is now seldom seen in children, adolescents or young adults because of prompt treatment of respiratory infections and because of immunization programmes. It is not often seen in the middle-aged because they are likely to have had the bronchiectatic area(s) resected 20 or more years ago. It is, however, not very uncommon in the elderly, although often labelled as 'chronic bronchitis' for many years.

The possibility of bronchiectasis usually arises in the differential diagnosis of haemoptysis or a slowly resolving pneumonia.

### Bronchography

This is the only definitive investigation, but can hardly be justified in the elderly because a positive diagnosis will not influence therapy since resection is contra-indicated and postural drainage should be advised for chronic productive cough in any case. Even to exclude neoplasm, the investigation is not justified in this age group.

### Tomography

This may be helpful in showing patency or narrowing of larger bronchi, solid lesions, fibrotic shadowing, atelectatic areas or multiple small ring shadows.

**Complications**
These include pneumonia (often recurring in the same site), pleurisy, effusion, haemoptysis, brain abscess and amyloidosis.

**Treatment**
This consists of antimicrobial therapy for acute exacerbations, postural drainage, and, in selected cases with copious persistent sputum, long-term antimicrobial therapy. Anabolic steroids may be helpful in restoring positive nitrogen balance.

## 2. SARCOIDOSIS

Although rare in the elderly, sarcoidosis is not unknown as a cause of diffuse pulmonary opacities (sometimes with hilar adenopathy) and breathlessness.

In the subacute stage the Kveim test is usually positive, but in the chronic stage with insidious onset which is more common in the elderly the Kveim test may be negative.

Other manifestations that may be noted are skin plaques, and posterior uveitis, in particular. Bone cysts are *not* seen unless there are overlying skin lesions. Hypercalciuria is more often noted than hypercalcaemia.

Biopsy of some accessible tissue is crucial to definite diagnosis.

Acute manifestations are usually suppressed by corticosteroid administration but established fibrosis is not affected.

## 3. SPONTANEOUS PNEUMOTHORAX

This is not infrequently a cause of sudden death in elderly bronchitics. The chief manifestations are pleuritic pain, increased dyspnoea, cyanosis and shock. The characteristic clinical findings are weak or absent breath-sounds and hyperresonant percussion note. Chest X-ray shows a lung edge separated from the bony cage of the thorax by a clear area.

The differential diagnosis is from myocardial infarction (ECG, enzymes), pulmonary infarction (*see* Chapter Nine) and other causes of pleurisy (*see* Chapter Ten).

Treatment consists of oxygen-enriched air, bronchodilators, antimicrobials and if there is much respiratory distress a tube (leading to an underwater seal) may be inserted to relieve the pressure.

## 4. DIFFUSE FIBROSING ALVEOLITIS

About 50 per cent of cases first develop symptoms in the seventh decade.

### Aetiology

*A.* Extrinsic allergic alveolitis (chronic form)
  i. Due to a variety of antigens, e.g., aspergillosis, bird fancier's lung, farmer's lung, etc.
  ii. Serum precipitins against relevant antigen

*B.* Drugs, e.g., hexamethonium, busulphan, chlorambucil

*C.* Collagenoses, e.g., rheumatoid disease, systemic sclerosis

*D.* Possible genetic factor—high incidence in twins

### Functional Effects

1. Restrictive spirometric pattern
2. Impaired diffusion
3. Hypoxaemia on exercise; eventually hypoxaemia at rest
4. Reduced compliance ('stiff' lungs)

### Clinical Features

1. Severe dyspnoea early; cyanosis later; cough with secondary infection

2. Clubbing frequent; hypertrophic pulmonary osteo-arthropathy may occur
3. Loud coarse crackles on auscultation
4. Cor pulmonale eventually
5. Serum ANF and/or RA tests may be positive

**Chest X-ray**

1. Chronic form: diffuse fine mottling more marked in lower zones with later a 'honeycomb' appearance
2. Subacute form: appears similar to bronchopneumonia

**Differential Diagnosis**

1. Chronic: lymphangitic carcinomatosis, alveolar cell carcinoma, tuberculosis and sarcoidosis may all give similar picture
2. Subacute: as for chronic plus pulmonary oedema, bronchopneumonia, pulmonary alveolar proteinosis and multiple pulmonary infarcts all have to be considered

**Treatment**

The only treatment likely to have any effect in fibrosing alveolitis and most of the differential diagnoses (except tuberculosis, infarction and bronchopneumonia) is the use of a corticosteroid. For this reason lung biopsy would be only of academic interest at any age and certainly unjustifiable in the elderly.

## 5. RHEUMATOID DISEASE

This may produce a number of intrathoracic lesions:

*A*. Pleurisy and effusion
*B*. Diffuse fibrosing alveolitis
*C*. Caplan's syndrome (lung nodules on a pneumoconiotic background)
*D*. Solitary lung or pleural nodules (resembling neoplasms)

*E*. Pulmonary infiltrations and pleuropericarditis
*F*. Pulmonary arterial disease

**Treatment**—corticosteroid

## 6. SYSTEMIC LUPUS ERYTHEMATOSUS

Uncommon in the elderly.

*A*. Pericarditis and pleurisy and often effusion
*B*. 'Pneumonia' and atelectases (due to change in surfactant?)
*C*. Dyspnoea without obvious X-ray changes
*D*. X-ray may show:
   i. Effusion
   ii. Atelectases
   iii. Micronodular shadowing
   iv. Oedema
   v. Fibrosing alveolitis
*E*. Serum may show positive ANF test and LE cells

**Treatment**—corticosteroid

## 7. SYSTEMIC SCLEROSIS

Lung lesions occur in 50 per cent of cases.

*A*. Dyspnoea and cough (may be mucoid sputum)
*B*. If severe—basal crackles and cyanosis
*C*. Secondary infection common
*D*. Aspiration pneumonia from overspill from affected oesophagus
*E*. Pulmonary oedema may occur secondary to:
   i. Hypertension (secondary to renal involvement)
   ii. Cardiac involvement
*F*. Skin lesions mandatory to diagnosis
*G*. Restrictive spirometric pattern with impaired diffusion

**Treatment**—corticosteroid

*Section 3*

# Special Problems

*Chapter Thirteen*

# Symptomatic Management

## 1. HAEMOPTYSIS

*A.* Associated with acute infection—appropriate antimicrobial

*B.* Associated with pulmonary infarction—anti-coagulant, etc.

*C.* Associated with carcinoma:

- i. If severe or distressing—cytotoxic or radio-therapy
- ii. Ethamsylate sometimes effective

*D.* Associated with bronchiectasis:

- i. Antimicrobial
- ii. Postural drainage
- iii. Ethamsylate

*E.* Associated with tuberculosis—antituberculous drugs

*F.* Associated with cardiac lesions—treat left-heart failure

*G.* No obvious cause

- i. Ethamsylate
- ii. Repeat X-ray in 4–6 weeks
- iii. Further follow-up as situation dictates

## 2. DYSPNOEA

### A. Cardiac

i. *Paroxysmal nocturnal dyspnoea* (pulmonary oedema)

*a.* Emergency treatment with intravenous

frusemide and intravenous aminophylline may give rapid relief

*b.* A phenothiazine will relieve anxiety

*c.* Oxygen therapy should be given (if definitely no lung disease 100 per cent may be used)

*d.* If not previously digitalized intravenous digoxin can be given, otherwise oral dosage continued or slightly increased

*e.* Maintenance therapy with oral diuretic plus potassium or potassium-sparing agent, digoxin and a neutral xanthine suppository (at night)

*f.* Sleep propped-up

ii. *Exertional dyspnoea*

Diuretic, digoxin and xanthine in various combinations will usually improve exercise tolerance to a variable degree.

**B. Respiratory**

i. *Acute asthma*

*a.* β-2 adrenergic stimulating bronchodilator is mainstay of treatment, e.g., terbutaline or salbutamol; by pressurized aerosol or orally

*b.* A xanthine, e.g., proxyphylline, may be used as an alternative or additional measure; oral, rectal or intravenous routes effective

*c.* Oxygen—acute asthmatics are hypoxaemic!

*d.* Failure of response to above—status asthmaticus for which corticosteroid therapy is mandatory (adequate dose must be used—60 mg. prednisone (or equivalent) in the first 24 hours)

ii. *Chronic reversible obstruction*

*a.* β-2 adrenergic stimulator

*b.* Xanthine

*c.* Corticosteroids in some cases: beclomethasone aerosol is effective maintenance therapy with much smaller dosage of corticosteroid, hence much less likelihood of side-effects.

iii. *Acute infections*
  *a.* Appropriate antimicrobial
  *b.* Temporary use of bronchodilators
iv. *Restrictive disease*
  Corticosteroid may give some relief
v. *Irreversible*
  When no response to β-2 adrenergic stimulator, xanthine or corticosteroid the inevitable should be accepted and a simple tranquillizer given

**C. Mixed Cardiac and Respiratory**
i. Acute: xanthines are safe in both cardiac and respiratory illness
ii. Various factors must be treated on their merits (*see* Chapter Fourteen).

## 3. COUGH

*A.* Treat causes (Chapter Two) whenever possible.

*B.* Unproductive cough in itself warrants relief with codeine phosphate, pholcodine or noscapine.

*C.* Productive cough may warrant some degree of suppression when it is seriously affecting sleep, especially where prognosis is poor, e.g., an advanced elderly bronchitic.

*D.* Cough due to carcinoma merits suppression whether productive or not; diamorphine hydrochloride remains the best available cough suppressant in addition to its pain-relieving function.

*E.* All cough suppressants are likely to cause constipation; it seems logical in the elderly to give a suitable laxative concurrently.

## 4. EXPECTORATION

*A.* Postural drainage is probably the most helpful aid to expectoration; unfortunately elderly patients often cannot tolerate the procedure.

*B.* Traditional 'expectorant' mixtures contain guiac, ipecachuana or ammonium chloride as the 'active' ingredient; there is no convincing evidence that they are effective.

*C.* A more scientific approach has been to employ 'mucolytic agents' of which bromhexine, cysteine derivatives and proteolytic [sic] enzymes appear to have reduced sputum viscosity in some cases; evidence concerning clinical effectiveness is conflicting and on the whole unconvincing; one feature that seems to have been overlooked in all studies is that a small gobbet of very thick sputum may cause enormous distress.

*D.* A microaerosol of warmed water has been shown to be the most effective means of reducing sputum viscosity, but again subjective improvement is variable; where a suitable nebulization apparatus is not available, steam inhalations are often helpful.

## 5. CHEST PAIN

### A. Angina

i. A major advance in therapy has taken place in recent years with the introduction of β adrenergic blockers; some hazard lies in the possibility of provoking, or worsening already existing, cardiac failure by their negative inotropic effect; the best to date appears to be oxprenolol (average dose 120–240 mg. daily in divided doses, may be increased to 480 mg. if required); care also has to be taken in asthmatics as bronchospasm occasionally may be induced
ii. Glyceryl trinitrate has stood the test of time and may be used in conjunction with a beta blocker if necessary
iii. So-called 'long-acting' nitrates have not stood up to critical examination

iv. Other drugs claimed to be useful may be of value in individual cases, e.g., verapamil, prenylamine
v. A tranquillizer is frequently required; chlodiazepoxide (15–30 mg. daily in divided doses) or diazepam (6–15 mg. daily in divided doses) is generally satisfactory

**B. Myocardial Infarction**

i. Morphine (10 mg. in the elderly) is still the most effective, but various morphine derivatives or synthetic analogues may be used in individual cases; care must be taken if there is concurrent respiratory disease; in which situation the respiratory depression can be counteracted by simultaneous administration of levallorphan
ii. Pentazocine may be sufficient in some patients with less severe pain
iii. Tranquillization usually helpful

**C. Pleurisy**

i. Paracetamol or dextropropoxyphene, alone or in combination, is safe and may suffice for pain relief
ii. Pentazocine may be used if above unsatisfactory
iii. Very severe pain may require morphine plus levallorphan
iv. Dihydrocodeinone to be avoided if any asthmatic tendency as it may provoke bronchospasm

**D. Carcinoma**

i. Pain may be from pleural or bony involvement
ii. It is usually necessary to progress through the range of the analgesics up to the powerful narcotics; undoubtedly the most effective drug is diamorphine hydrochloride
iii. In some cases radiotherapy or cytotoxic drugs may give relief

iv. Where facilities exist it is worth considering electrical cordotomy if narcotics cannot be tolerated or are refused

**E. Fractured Ribs**

i. Do not immobilize chest; this interferes with respiration and effective coughing thus leading to atelectasis infection, etc.
ii. Simple analgesics and local infiltration with local anaesthetic are generally effective

**F. Root Pain**

i. Simple analgesics
ii. Spinal support
iii. Phenylbutazone often very helpful in pain from collapsed vertebrae from osteoporosis

**G. Hiatus Hernia**

i. Antacids may be helpful, especially when combined with a mucosal local anaesthetic (oxethazaine)
ii. Patient should sleep propped-up, eat standing up or at least walk around after eating
iii. A preparation containing alginic acid plus antacids may be useful in some patients

*Chapter Fourteen*

# Respiratory Disease associated with other Systemic Diseases

## 1. RESPIRATORY AND CARDIAC DISEASE

A COMMON difficulty in elderly patients is that cardiac and respiratory disease may exist side by side as

*A*. Cardiac and respiratory disease of separate aetiologies

*B*. Cardiac complications of respiratory disease or

*C*. Respiratory symptoms secondary to cardiac disease

The main problem is usually whether dyspnoea is primarily cardiac or respiratory in origin.

In both cardiac and respiratory disease, dyspnoea of any severity, constant or paroxysmal, nocturnal as well as diurnal, may occur. A history of dyspnoea on recumbency necessitating sleeping propped up (orthopnoea) is characteristic of left-sided heart failure. Some chronic bronchitics, however, give a similar type of history which can easily be confused with true paroxysmal nocturnal dyspnoea. Careful questioning may be required to reveal that in fact these patients either start to cough when they lie flat or are woken by coughing, which is then followed by the sensation of dyspnoea. The problem is further confounded by the occasional elderly asthmatic who has nocturnal attacks of bronchial asthma; often these attacks are related to thermal changes.

A history of cough and sputum on most days for three consecutive months for at least two successive years indicates chronic bronchitis, but this does not preclude co-existence cardiac disease. On the other hand, absence of such a history is strong evidence against chronic bronchitis, especially if there is past evidence of cardiac disease, e.g., a history of myocardial infarction.

Chest pain also may be a trap for the unwary for the patient with chronic airways obstruction may describe a sensation of tightness across the chest or around the costal margin very similar to the constricting pain described by some anginal sufferers, often occurring on exertion in the same way also. In addition it is not at all uncommon for chronic bronchitics to complain of sub-sternal pain (the sensation being frequently called a soreness) but this is generally associated with coughing.

An electrocardiogram may show evidence of myocardial ischaemia or left ventricular hypertrophy (i.e., S in $V_1$ + R in $V_5$ greater than 35 mV.; T inversion of 'hypertrophy' type is supporting evidence as are T inversion in other leads, left-bundle branch block, or left axis deviation). Exercise may be required to elicit ischaemic changes in some patients. An alternative to exercise in producing such changes is the intravenous administration of isoprenaline (which increases myocardial oxygen requirements). In chronic lung disease the electrocardiogram will show evidence of right ventricular hypertrophy (i.e., dominant R waves over right ventricular leads $V_4R$, $V_3R$, $V_1$ and sometimes $V_2$, with dominant S wave in $V_5$; additional but not pathognomic signs are right-axis deviation, T inversion over right ventricular leads and leads 3 and AVF, right-bundle branch block or pulmonary type-P waves). Some electrocardiograms will show evidence of both right and left ventricular hypertrophy or right ventricular hypertrophy plus ischaemic changes.

Measurement of $FEV_1$ and FVC will demonstrate the presence or absence of expiratory airways obstruction and repetition after the administration of a bronchodilator will indicate the degree of reversibility (if any). A restrictive pattern may be found in cardiac failure as well as in infiltrative or fibrotic lung disease. Blood gas measurements can prove helpful. Hypoxaemia is likely to be found both in chronic respiratory and cardiac disease, but a normal or low arterial $P_{CO_2}$ virtually excludes cardiac failure secondary to chronic pulmonary disease. On the other hand, a raised $P_{CO_2}$ which indicates generalized underventilation does not preclude the possibility of independent cardiac disease in a patient with chronic pulmonary disease.

Chest X-rays may show the presence of intrapulmonary disease, congestive changes, effusions or cardiac enlargement and will have to be interpreted in the light of clinical and other findings. A normal heart outline, of course, is a point against the condition being primarily cardiac.

Another situation which may produce some confusion is where a patient with chronic pulmonary disease has basal crackles and right-heart failure. The question then arises whether or not he has left-heart failure also. This problem is further compounded by the realization that some impairment of left ventricular function has been demonstrated by modern techniques in emphysema *per se*! Even after judicious assessment of all the evidence, the issue may remain in doubt in the individual patient.

Similar considerations pertain to the simultaneous occurrence of hypertension and chronic pulmonary disease. The mere occurrence of a raised mean blood-pressure does not in itself prove that the cardiac failure is hypertensive in origin. Nevertheless, it is not uncommon for bronchitis to be superimposed on hypertensive heart failure or for recurrent attacks of pulmonary oedema with expectoration of frothy sputum to be misdiagnosed as chronic bronchitis. Electrocardiography and response to specific therapy are helpful pointers to correct diagnosis.

Yet another potent source of difficulty is the occurrence of respiratory symptoms in a patient with established cardiac disease, e.g., pleurisy in a patient recovering from myocardial infarction, sudden onset of dyspnoea at rest in hypertensive heart disease, or cough with blood-stained sputum in a patient with arteriosclerotic cardiac failure.

Such manifestations are often thought initially to be pneumonic; indeed the chest X-ray may actually be reported as showing 'consolidation' or 'an area of pneumonitis [sic]', and there may be fever and leucocytosis. Some of these episodes are infective but many of them really are pulmonary infarcts. Maintaining a high index of suspicion helps in diagnosing such incidents for it is clearly desirable to recognize this state of affairs at the earliest possible moment. The investigation and treatment has already been discussed in an earlier chapter (*see* Chapter Nine).

Management of combined respiratory and cardiac disease consists of judicious balance of treatment directed at both, with antibiotics, controlled oxygen, selective $\beta$-2 bronchodilators, diuretics and, if indicated, corticosteroids and digoxin.

## 2. RESPIRATORY AND CEREBROVASCULAR DISEASE

This combination is common since bronchopneumonia is a frequent complication of cerebrovascular catastrophes and often the proximate cause of death.

The hemiplegic unconscious patient may be unable to cough, thus retaining in his bronchi secretions which are likely to become infected. In addition, lying prone impairs venous return to the right heart thus leading to pulmonary congestion.

If such a patient is nursed in a semi-recumbent position gravity will produce increased congestion of the lung bases (which even in the normal have a relatively greater perfusion than the mid-zones or apices), with subsequent exudation of fluid which in time becomes infected so producing the so-called 'hypostatic pneumonia'.

A further complication is that the immobility of such patients renders them likely to develop venous thrombosis and pulmonary embolism.

In addition the development of a cerebrovascular incident in a patient with pre-existing chronic pulmonary disease renders the chances of all these complications much higher.

The occurrence of cerebral and respiratory disease in the same patient should always arouse the suspicion of an intrapulmonary neoplasm with cerebral secondary and in a known bronchiectatic cerebral symptoms should raise the possibility of brain abscess.

Management of respiratory complications of cerebral disease is primarily aimed at prevention, i.e., frequent changes of position, passive movements of limbs, repeated examination of lung bases for crackles, frequent examination of legs for signs of thrombosis, elevation of foot of bed, attention to pressure areas and careful attention to the state of fluid balance (avoiding both under- and over-hydration).

Treatment of established complications follows the methods outlined in previous chapters. There is no evidence that prophylactic antibiotics are of any value. Indeed it is quite common to find that a terminal bronchopneumonia fails to respond to such therapy, probably because the stagnation factor leading to a subacute form of pulmonary oedema has been overlooked. In fact it is probably more logical to use diuretics as a prophylactic measure although there is no scientific proof that this is effective.

## 3. RESPIRATORY DISEASE AND MENTAL STATE

There are a number of ways in which respiratory disease may affect a patient's mental state.

### A. Hypoxaemia

Leading to cerebral hypoxia, this may produce clouding of consciousness, paranoia or anxiety (often agitated).

### B. Hypercapnia

This leads to drowsiness, impaired consciousness and eventual coma.

### C. Chronic Lung Disease

Like any other chronic illness, this may produce depression, anxiety or both. Relief of depression in such patients often leads to improved respiration.

### D. Asthma

This may be precipitated by anxiety and in turn may produce anxiety thus triggering off a vicious cycle. Tranquillizers are often helpful in this situation.

### E. Recurrent Chest Infections

This may produce toxi-confusional states which recover as the infection subsides. When such episodes recur frequently the use of long-term continuous antimicrobial therapy should be seriously considered.

## 4. RESPIRATORY AND NEUROLOGICAL DISEASE

Carcinoma of bronchus may present with or develop a variety of neurological syndromes which have been described earlier (*see* Chapter Six). Brain abscess may occur as a complication of bronchiectasis. Patients with motor neuron disease or myasthenia gravis may develop ventilatory insufficiency, as may patients with ascending myelitis or poliomyelitis.

## 5. RESPIRATORY AND GASTROINTESTINAL DISEASE

There is said to be an increased risk of developing pulmonary tuberculosis in patients who have been subjected to gastrectomy. The evidence is not very convincing. Similarly the evidence suggesting that there is an increased incidence of peptic ulceration in emphysema/chronic bronchitis is rather tenuous, especially as both are common in the elderly. Peptic ulcer is of importance in relation to the use of corticosteroids in some lung conditions because of the risk of haemorrhage.

Certain systemic diseases with major pulmonary manifestations may have associated gastro-intestinal dysfunction, e.g., malabsorption in tuberculosis, sarcoidosis or systemic sclerosis. Diarrhoea may result from antibiotic therapy destroying the bacterial flora of the gut. Achalasia of the cardia may permit reflux oesophagitis with eventual 'dysphagic pneumonitis' from overspill. Rupture of the oesophagus may produce pleural effusion, oesophago-pleural fistula or mediastinal emphysema.

## 6. RESPIRATORY AND SKELETAL DISEASE

Ankylosing spondylitis may be associated with a non-specific upper lobe fibrosis (not necessarily related to previous radiotherapy). Some cases have also been described with upper-lobe mycetoma.

Bronchial carcinoma may be complicated by secondary deposits in vertebrae or ribs.

Cervical spondylosis and thoracic osteoarthritis are common in the elderly and may complicate any lung disease, and enter into the differential diagnosis of chest pain.

## 7. RESPIRATORY AND ENDOCRINE DISEASE

In diabetes mellitus there is an increased susceptibility to tuberculosis and respiratory infection in general, and conversely such infections cause deterioration in control of the diabetes.

Addison's disease may be associated with pulmonary tuberculosis, and hypothyroidism may occur in patients who have had para-amino salicylic acid as part of their antituberculous therapy.

The endocrine manifestations of bronchial carcinoma have been described earlier (*see* Chapter Six).

## 8. RESPIRATORY DISEASE AND ANAEMIA

Apart from anaemias as a complication of pulmonary tuberculosis or bronchial carcinoma, any anaemia may worsen the functional disturbance in any serious pulmonary disease. This is because the oxygen capacity and content are reduced, as shown in Table 4.

Table 4—Oxygen capacity and content in respiratory disease and anaemia

| Haemoglobin (g. per cent) | $O_2$ capacity (ml. per cent) | $O_2$ saturation (per cent) | $O_2$ content (ml. per cent) |
|---|---|---|---|
| 15 | 20 | 95 | 19 |
| 15 | 20 | 60 | 12 |
| 9 | 12 | 95 | 11·4 |
| 9 | 12 | 60 | 7·2 |

*Chapter Fifteen*

# Adverse Effects of Drugs

## 1. GENERAL

*A.* Increased risk of toxicity in the elderly because:

i. Decreased lean body mass

ii. Multiple pathology tempts to polypharmacy

iii. Impaired functional reserve, especially renal and hepatic (creatinine clearance may be low despite normal serum creatinine and urea)

iv. Forgetfulness when self-medication required may lead to overdosage

## 2. ANTIMICROBIALS

*A.* May produce rashes and other hypersensitivity reactions (including pyrexia)

*B.* The most important toxic effects which may be produced are:

i. Cephaloridine—nephrotoxicity (rare)

ii. Chloramphenicol—blood dyscrasias

iii. Co-trimoxazole—gastric disturbances

iv. Colistin—nephrotoxicity

v. Ethambutol—optic neuritis (rare with 7 mg. per kg. body-weight dosage)

vi. Fusidic acid—gastric disturbances

vii. Gentamycin—ototoxicity

viii. Isoniazid—peripheral neoropathy, psychosis, thrombocytopenia (all rare with normal dosage of 200–300 mg. daily)

ix. Kanamycin—ototoxicity
x. Lincomycin—gastric disturbances
xi. Nalidixic acid—phototoxicity
xii. Neomycin—ototoxicity
xiii. Nitrofurantoin—gastric disturbances, exacerbation of renal failure
xiv. Novobiocin—thrombocytopenia
xv. Para-amino salicylic acid (PAS)—gastric disturbances, hypoprothrombinaemia, hypothyroidism, exfoliative dermatitis and hepatotoxicity
xvi. Polymixins—nephrotoxicity
xvii. Rifampicin—hepatotoxicity
xviii. Streptomycin—ototoxicity
xix. Sulphonamides—crystalluria, blood dyscrasias
xx. Tetracyclines—exacerbation of renal failure, phototoxicity

## 3. BRONCHODILATORS

*A*. *β-adrenergic stimulators* may produce:
i. Increased hypoxaemia
ii. Tachycardia
iii. Tremor

*B*. *Xanthines* may produce:
i. Nausea and vomiting
ii. Increased hypoxaemia
iii. Tachycardia
iv. Hypotension

## 4. CORTICOSTEROIDS may produce

*A*. Hypertension
*B*. Sodium and water retention
*C*. Potassium depletion

*D*. Peptic ulceration
*E*. Diabetes mellitus
*F*. Osteoporosis
*G*. Recrudescence of tuberculosis
*H*. Masking of infections
*I*. Skin ecchymoses
*J*. Psychosis
*K*. Cushingoid appearance
*L*. Increased tendency to venous thrombosis
*M*. Increased tendency to cataracts
*N*. Increased tendency to open angle glaucoma
*O*. Myopathy
*P*. Adrenal suppression

5. **PHENOTHIAZINES** may produce:
*A*. Potentiation of opiates and hypnotics
*B*. Lethargy
*C*. Parkinsonism
*D*. Hypotension
*E*. Hypothermia
*F*. Cholestatic jaundice
*G*. Photosensitivity
*H*. Increased constipation

6. **BENZODIAZEPINES** may produce:
*A*. Hypotension
*B*. Apnoea (when given intravenously)

7. **TRICYCLIC ANTI-DEPRESSANTS** may produce:
*A*. Hypotension
*B*. Drowsiness
*C*. Anticholinergic effects

## 8. DIURETICS

*A. Thiazides, frusemide, ethacrynic acid* may produce:
- i. Hypokalaemia and hyponatraemia
- ii. Hypotension
- iii. Precipitation of incontinence of urine
- iv. Increased tendency to venous thrombosis
- v. Hyperuricaemia and gout
- vi. Unmasking of latent diabetes
- vii. Phototoxicity

*B. Triamterine, amiloride and spironolactone* may produce:
- i. Hyperkalaemia

## 9. OPIATES, BARBITURATES AND OTHER HYPNOTICS may produce:

- *A.* Respiratory depression (except benzoctamine which stimulates)
- *B.* Potentiation of antihypertensive drugs
- *C.* Mental depression
- *D.* Phototoxicity
- *E.* Increased effects in the presence of
  - i. Hypoxaemia
  - ii. Anaemia
  - iii. Hypothyroidism

## 10. β-ADRENERGIC BLOCKERS may produce:

- *A.* Increased airways resistance
- *B.* Precipitation of cardiac failure
- *C.* Bradycardia
- *D.* Masking of hypoglycaemia due to antidiabetic drugs
- *E.* Mental depression

11. **DIGOXIN** may produce:

*A.* Cardiac arrythmias
*B.* Gastric disturbances
*C.* Toxi-confusional states
*D.* Increased toxicity in presence of hypokalaemia
*E.* A type of 'acute abdomen'

12. **α-METHYL DOPA** may produce:

*A.* Severe hypotension
*B.* Drowsiness
*C.* Mental depression
*D.* Sodium and water retention
*E.* Haemolytic anaemia
*F.* Unfavourable interaction with tricyclic antidepressants

13. **CARBENOXOLONE AND PHENYLBUTAZONE** may produce:

*A.* Sodium and water retention

14. **DRUG INTERACTIONS**

*A.* *Impairment of absorption*
i. Tetracycline—by ferrous sulphate
ii. Barbiturates }
iii. Salicylates } by alkalis
iv. Sulphonamides }

*B.* *Competition for serum protein-binding*
i. Phenylbutazone enhances effects of antidiabetic sulphonamides
ii. Phenylbutazone enhances effects of anticoagulants
iii. Aspirin enhances effects of anticoagulants

*C. Enzyme depression*

Mono-amine oxidase inhibitor drugs enhance effects of:

i. Sympathomimetic amines
ii. Alcohol
iii. Pethidene
iv. Barbiturates

*D. Enzyme induction*

Barbiturates reduce effects of:

i. Anticoagulants
ii. Phenytoin
iii. Phenylbutazone

# Diagnosis of 500 consecutive Hospital Cases

Diagnosis on discharge between 1 January, 1969, and 31 December, 1970, of 513 patients aged 65 or over admitted with respiratory symptoms

| | Male | | Female | |
|---|---|---|---|---|
| | No. | Per cent | No. | Per cent |
| Exacerbations of chronic bronchitis | 106 | 37·1 | 56 | 24·7 |
| Cardiovascular disease | 59 | 20·6 | 85 | 37·4 |
| Bronchopneumonias | 37 | 11·9 | 39 | 17·2 |
| Bronchial carcinoma | 18 | 6·3 | 7 | 3·1 |
| Pulmonary heart disease | 13 | 4·5 | 4 | 1·8 |
| Acute bronchitis | 10 | 3·5 | 3 | 1·3 |
| Pneumococcal lobar pneumonias | 9 | 3·1 | 4 | 1·8 |
| Pulmonary fibrosis | 9 | 3·1 | 7 | 3·1 |
| Pulmonary infarction | 7 | 2·4 | 3 | 1·3 |
| Bronchial asthma | 4 | 1·4 | 4 | 1·8 |
| Spontaneous pneumothorax | 4 | 1·4 | 0 | 0 |
| Pleurisy | 2 | 0·7 | 2 | 0·9 |
| Bronchiectasis | 2 | 0·7 | 5 | 2·2 |
| Fractured ribs | 1 | 0·3 | 0 | 0 |
| Lung abscess | 1 | 0.3 | 0 | 0 |
| Lymphatic leukaemia | 0 | 0 | 1 | 0.4 |
| Other lung neoplasm | 0 | 0 | 1 | 0·4 |
| Laryngeal neoplasm | 0 | 0 | 1 | 0.4 |
| Sarcoidosis | 0 | 0 | 1 | 0·4 |
| Oesophageal neoplasm | 0 | 0 | 1 | 0·4 |
| Other respiratory illnesses (e.g., influenza, haemoptysis of unknown cause, etc.) | 4 | 1·4 | 3 | 1·3 |
| Total | 286 | 100 | 227 | 100 |

*Appendix B*

# Selected Bibliography


BRAIN, Lord (1963), The neurological complications of neoplasms, *Lancet*, **1**, 179.

BURROWS, B., FLETCHER, C. M., HEARD, B. E., JONES, N. L., and WOOTLIFF, J. S. (1966), 'The emphysematous and bronchitic types of chronic airways obstruction', *Ibid.*, **1**, 830.

CAIRD, F. I., and AKHTAR, A. J. (1972), 'Chronic respiratory disease in the elderly', *Thorax*, **27**, 764.

CROFTON, J., and DOUGLAS, A. (1969), *Respiratory Diseases.* Oxford and Edinburgh: Blackwell Scientific.

COTES, J. E. (1965), *Lung Function. Assessment and Application in Medicine.* Oxford and Edinburgh: Blackwell Scientific.

Editorial (1968), 'Endocrine disorders associated with carcinoma', *Br. med. J.*, **2**, 5.

EXTON-SMITH, A. N., and CORLESS, D. (1965), 'Respiratory disorders in the elderly', *Practitioner*, **195**, 755.

FULLERTON, J. M., and DYER, L. (1965), 'Unsuspected tuberculosis in the aged', *Tubercle, Lond.*, **46**, 193.

GILSON, J. C. (1966), 'The ageing lung', in *Medicine in Old Age* (ed. AGATE, D.). London: Pitman.

GRIMBY, G., and SÖDERHOLM, B. (1962), 'Energy expenditure of men in different age groups during level walking and bicycle ergometry', *Scand. J. clin. lab. Invest.*, **14**, 321.

HARANGHY, L., MARK, I., RACZ, P., SZEMENYEI, K., MESZAROS, A., and FLEISCHMANN, I. (1960), 'Pathology of tuberculosis in old age', *Geront. clin.*, **2**, 18.

HARRIS, L. (1973) 'The discriminatory value of the single-breath carbon monoxide diffusion coefficient (*k*CO) in chronic airways obstruction', *Bull. Physio-path. Resp.* **9**, 473.

—— *Clinical Respiratory Physiology.* Bristol: John Wright. To be published.

HEMINGWAY, A., POCKOCK, D., and SHORT, J. J. (1956), 'Variations of basal respiration with age', *J. Chron. Dis.*, **3**, 301.

HIGGS, B. E., CLODE, M., MCHARDY, G. J. R., JONES, N. L., and CAMPBELL, E. J. M. (1966), 'Changes in ventilation, gas exchange and circulation during exercise in normal subjects', *Clin. Sci.*, **32**, 329.

HOWELL, T. H. (1965), 'Problems of respiratory disease in old age', *J. Indian med. Prof.*, **11**, 5206.

JONES, N. L., CAMPBELL, E. J. M., MCHARDY, G. J. R., HIGGS, B. E., and CLODE, M. (1967), 'The estimation of carbon dioxide pressure of mixed venous blood during exercise', *Clin. Sci.*, **32**, 311.

LAWS, J. W., and HEARD, B. E. (1962), 'Emphysema and the chest film: a retrospective radiological and pathological study', *Br. J. Radiol.*, **35**, 419.

MCHARDY, G. J. R. (1967), Paper 939, Tables 32/8 to 32/13, *Clin. Sci.*, obtainable from Librarian, Royal Society of Medicine.

MCKEOWN, F. (1965), *Pathology of the Aged.* London: Butterworths.

MAYER, E., BLAZSIK, C., and RAPPAPORT, I. (1958), 'Emphysema and the lungs of the aged: a clinical study', *Dis. Chest*, **34**, 247.

MEDICAL RESEARCH COUNCIL (1965), 'Definition and classification of chronic bronchitis', *Lancet*, **1**, 775.

MONROE, R. T. (1951), *Diseases of Old Age.* Cambridge, Mass.: Harvard University Press.

OGILVIE, A. G. (1962), 'Pulmonary disease in the elderly', *Practitioner*, **188**, 725.

PIERCE, J. A., and EBERT, R. V. (1958), 'The elastic properties of the lungs in the aged', *J. Lab. clin. Med.*, **51**, 63.

REID, L. (1967), *The Pathology of Emphysema.* London: Lloyd Luke.

RYAN, S. F., VINCENT, T. N., MITCHELL, R. S., FILLEY, G. F., and DART, G. (1963), 'Ductectasia, an asymptomatic pulmonary change related to age', *Med. Thorac.*, **22**, 81.

SCADDING, J. G. (1952), 'Chronic lung disease with diffuse nodular or reticular radiographic shadows', *Tubercle. Lond.*, **33**, 352.

SHOCK, N. W., and YUNGST, M. J. (1955), 'Age changes in basal respiratory measurements and metabolism in males', *J. Gerontol.*, **10**, 31.
SIMON, G. (1971), *Principles of Chest X-ray Diagnosis*, 3rd ed. London: Butterworths.
—— PRIDE, N. B., JONES, N. L., and RAIMONDI, A. C. (1973), 'Relation between abnormalities in the chest radiograph and changes in pulmonary function in chronic bronchitis and emphysema', *Thorax*, **28**, 15.
TRAILL, R. R. (1962), 'Pulmonary tuberculosis in old age', *Geriatrics*, **17**, 179.
VAN GANSE, W. F., FERRIS, B. G., and COTES, J. E. (1972), 'Cigarette smoking and pulmonary diffusing capacity (transfer factor)', *Am. Rev. Resp. Dis.*, **105**, 30.
WOODFORD-WILLIAMS, E. (1966), 'Diagnosis and management of pneumonia in the aged', *Br. med. J.*, **1**, 467.

# Index

Printed in France by Amazon
Brétigny-sur-Orge, FR

51786463R00087